Anatomy and Physiology for Nurses
at a Glance

Anatomy and Physiology for Nurses
at a Glance

Ian Peate
Professor of Nursing
Head of School
School of Health Studies
Gibraltar

Muralitharan Nair
Independent Nursing Consultant
England

Series Editor: Ian Peate

WILEY Blackwell

Registered Office

John Wiley & Sons, Ltd, The Atrium, Southern Gate, Chichester, West Sussex, PO19 8SQ, UK

Editorial Offices

9600 Garsington Road, Oxford, OX4 2DQ, UK

The Atrium, Southern Gate, Chichester, West Sussex, PO19 8SQ, UK

350 Main Street, Malden, MA 02148-5020, USA

For details of our global editorial offices, for customer services and for information about how to apply for permission to reuse the copyright material in this book please see our website at www.wiley.com/wiley-blackwell

Library of Congress Cataloging-in-Publication Data

Peate, Ian, author.

Anatomy and physiology for nurses at a glance / Ian Peate, Muralitharan Nair.

    p. ; cm.

  Includes bibliographical references and index.

  ISBN 978-1-118-74631-8 (paper)

I. Nair, Muralitharan, author.   II. Title.

[DNLM: 1. Anatomy–Nurses' Instruction.   2. Physiological Phenomena–Nurses' Instruction.   QS 4]

  QP38

  612–dc23

                                        2014032708

A catalogue record for this book is available from the British Library.

Wiley also publishes its books in a variety of electronic formats. Some content that appears in print may not be available in electronic books.

Cover image: PASIEKA/SCIENCE PHOTO LIBRARY

Set in 9.5/11.5pt Minion by SPi Publisher Services, Pondicherry, India

Printed and bound in Singapore by Markono Print Media Pte Ltd

1   2015

Contents

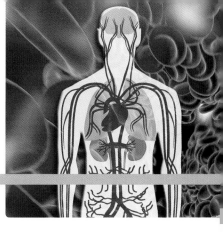

Part 1 — Foundations 1

Part 2 — The nervous system 19

Part 3 — The heart and vascular system 33

Part 4 — The respiratory system 49

Part 5 — The gastrointestinal tract 59

Appendices

Preface

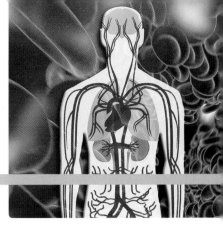

In order to care effectively for people (sick or well) the nurse has to have an understanding and insight into anatomy and physiology.

The human body is composed of organic and inorganic molecules that are organised at a variety of structural levels; despite this an individual should be seen and treated in a holistic manner. If the nurse is to provide appropriate and timely care, it is essential that they can recognise illness, deliver effective treatment and refer appropriately with the person at the centre of all they do.

Nurses are required to demonstrate a sound knowledge of anatomy and physiology with the intention of providing safe and effective nursing care. This is often assessed as a part of a programme of study. The overall aim of this concise text is to provide an overview of anatomy and physiology and the related biological sciences that can help to develop your practical caring skills and improve your knowledge with the aim of you becoming a caring, kind and compassionate nurse. It is anticipated that you will be able to deliver increasingly complex care for the people you care for when you understand how the body functions.

This text provides you with the opportunity to apply the content to the care of people. As you begin to appreciate how people respond or adapt to pathophysiological changes and stressors you will be able to understand that people (regardless of age) have specific biological needs.

The integration and application of evidence-based theory to practice is a key component of effective and safe health care. This goal cannot be achieved without an understanding of anatomy and physiology.

Living systems can be expressed from the very smallest level; the chemical level, atoms, molecules and the chemical bonds connecting atoms provide the structure upon which living activity is based. The smallest unit of life is the cell. Tissue is a group of cells that are alike, performing a common function. Organs are groups of different types of tissues working together to carry out a specific activity. Two or more organs working together to carry out a particular activity is described as a system. Another system that possesses the characteristics of living things is an organism, with the capacity to obtain and process energy, the ability to react to changes in the environment and to reproduce.

Anatomy is associated with the function of a living organism and as such it is almost always inseparable from physiology. Physiology is the science dealing with the study of the function of cells, tissues, organs and organisms; it is the study of life.

This *At A Glance* provides you with structure and a comprehensive approach to anatomy and physiology.

Ian Peate
Muralitharan Nair

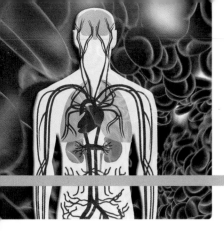

Abbreviations

ACTH	Adrenocorticotropic hormone		**HR**	Heart rate
ADH	Antidiuretic hormone		**K⁺**	Potassium
ANP	Atrial natriuretic peptide		**kPa**	Kilo Pascals
ANS	Autonomic nervous system		**Mg²⁺**	Magnesium
ATP	Adenosine triphosphate		**mmHg**	Millimetres of mercury
AV	Atrioventricular		**mRNA**	Messenger ribonucleic acid
BBB	Blood–brain barrier		**Na⁺**	Sodium
BP	Blood pressure		**NH3**	Ammonia
Ca²⁺	Calcium		**O₂**	Oxygen
CCK	Cholecystokinin		**PCA**	Posterior cerebral artery
CI	Chloride		**PCO₂**	Partial pressure of carbon dioxide
CNS	Central nervous system		**PO₂**	Partial pressure of oxygen
CRH	Corticotrophin releasing hormones		**PCT**	Proximal convoluted tubule
CSF	Cerebrospinal fluid		**pH**	A measure of the acidity or basicity of an aqueous solution
CO₂	Carbon dioxide			
CRC	Cardio-regulatory centre		**PNS**	Parasympathetic nervous system
CSF	Cerebrospinal fluid		**PRH**	Prolactin-releasing hormone
DNA	Deoxyribonucleic acid		**RBC**	Red blood cells
EPO	Erythropoietin		**RER**	Rough endoplasmic reticulum
FSH	Follicle-stimulating hormone		**SER**	Smooth endoplasmic reticulum
GH	Growth hormone		**RNA**	Ribonucleic acid
GHRIF	Growth hormone release-inhibiting factor		**tRNA**	Transfer ribonucleic acid
H⁺	Hydrogen		**rRNA**	Ribosomal ribonucleic acid
H₂O	Water		**SA**	Sinoatrial
Hb	Haemoglobin		**SNS**	Sympathetic nervous system
HCG	Human chorionic gonadotrophin		**TSH**	Thyroid-stimulating hormone
HCL	Hydrochloric acid		**WBC**	White blood cell

Acknowledgements

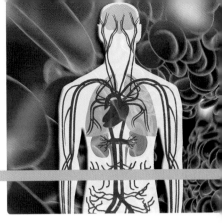

We acknowledge with thanks the use of material from other John Wiley & Sons publications:

Heffner L & Schust D (2014) *The Reproductive System at a Glance*, 4 edn. John Wiley & Sons, Ltd. Reproduced with permission of John Wiley & Sons, Ltd.

Jenkins G & Tortora GJ (2013) *Anatomy and Physiology: From Science to Life*, 3 edn. John Wiley & Sons, Ltd. Reproduced with permission of John Wiley & Sons, Ltd.

Mehta A & Hoffbrand V (2014) *Haematology at a Glance*, 4 edn. John Wiley & Sons, Ltd. Reproduced with permission of John Wiley & Sons, Ltd.

Nair, M & Peate I. (2013) *Fundamentals of Applied Pathophysiology* . John Wiley & Sons, Ltd. Reproduced with permission of John Wiley & Sons, Ltd.

Peate I & Nair M (2011) *Fundamentals of Anatomy and Physiology for Student Nurses*. John Wiley & Sons, Ltd. Reproduced with permission of John Wiley & Sons, Ltd.

Peate I, Wild K & Nair M (eds) (2014) *Nursing Practice: Knowledge and Care*. Reproduced with permission of John Wiley & Sons, Ltd.

Randall MD (ed.) (2014) *Medical Sciences at a Glance*. Reproduced with permission of John Wiley & Sons, Ltd.

Tortora GJ & Derrickson BH (2009) *Priniciples of Anatomy and Physiology*, 12 edn. Reproduced with permission of John Wiley & Sons, Ltd.

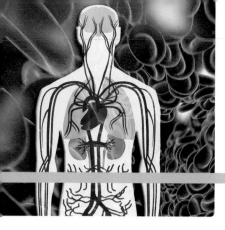

How to use your revision guide

Features contained within your revision guide

Each topic is presented in a double-page spread with clear, easy-to-follow diagrams supported by succinct explanatory text.

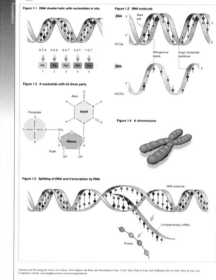

About the companion website

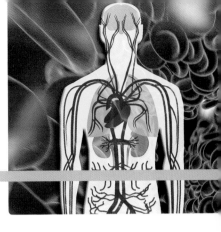

Don't forget to visit the companion website for this book:

www.ataglanceseries.com/nursing/anatomy

There you will find Interactive multiple choice questions designed
to enhance your learning.
Scan this QR code to visit the companion website:

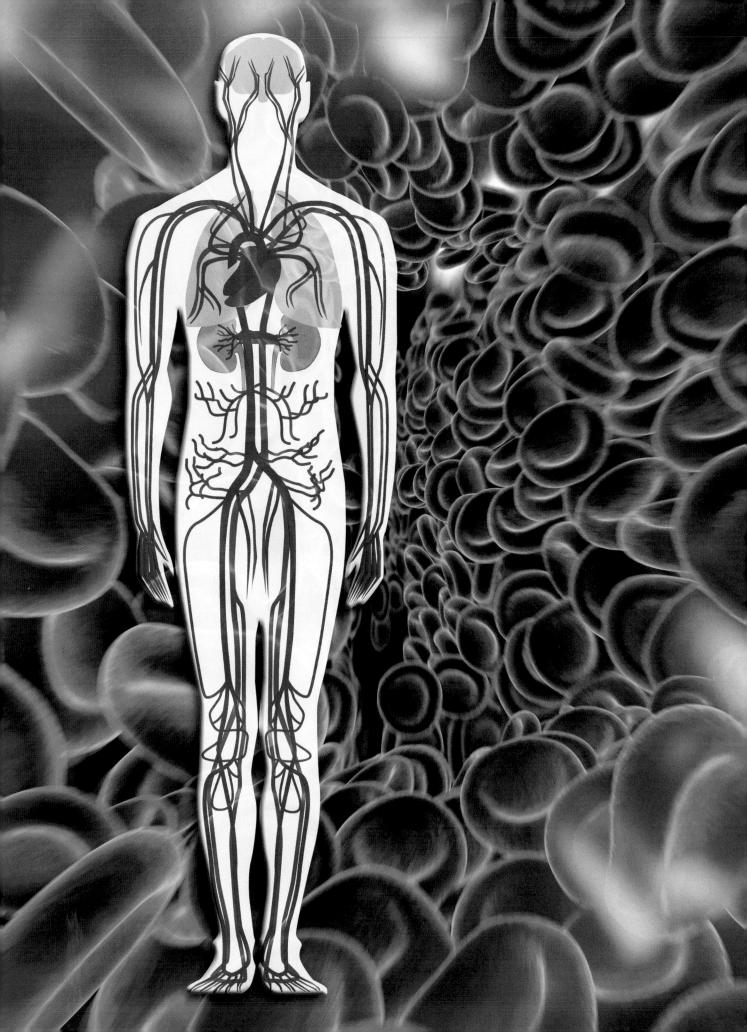

Foundations

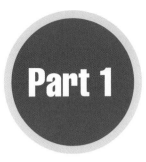

Part 1

Chapters

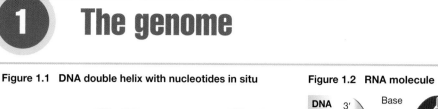

The genome

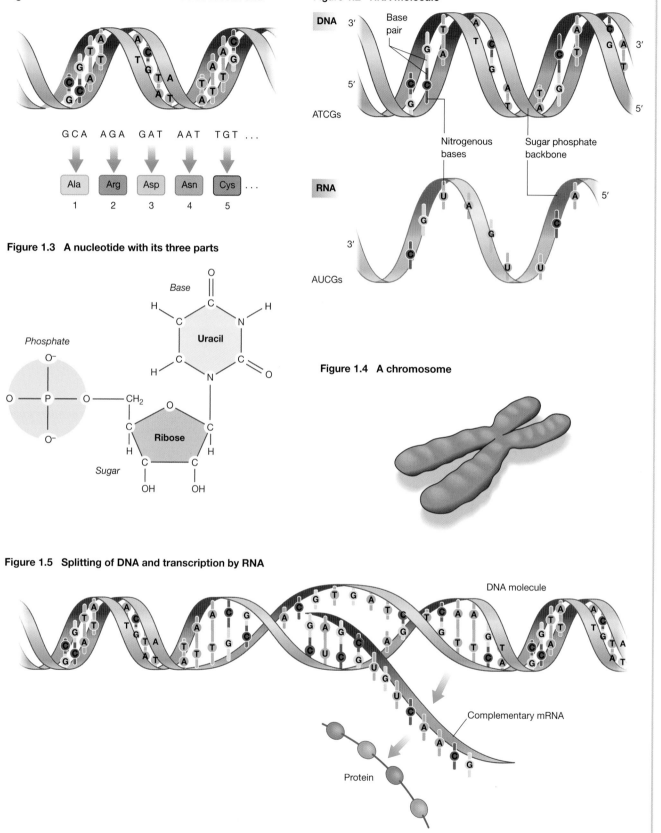

Figure 1.1 DNA double helix with nucleotides in situ

G C A   A G A   G A T   A A T   T G T ...

Ala	Arg	Asp	Asn	Cys	...
1	2	3	4	5	

Figure 1.3 A nucleotide with its three parts

Base

Phosphate

Uracil

Ribose

Sugar

Figure 1.2 RNA molecule

DNA

3′

Base pair

ATCGs

Nitrogenous bases

Sugar phosphate backbone

RNA

3′

AUCGs

Figure 1.4 A chromosome

Figure 1.5 Splitting of DNA and transcription by RNA

DNA molecule

Complementary mRNA

Protein

Anatomy and Physiology for Nurses at a Glance, First Edition. Ian Peate and Muralitharan Nair. © 2015 John Wiley & Sons, Ltd. Published 2015 by John Wiley & Sons, Ltd.
Companion website: www.ataglanceseries.com/nursing/anatomy

Genetics

Genetics is a fascinating subject and many diseases are linked to genes. Genes correspond to regions within DNA, a molecule composed of a chain of four different types of nucleotides – the sequence of these nucleotides is the genetic information organisms inherit. DNA naturally occurs in a double stranded form (double helix), with nucleotides on each strand complementary to each other (Figure 1.1). Each strand can act as a template for creating a new partner strand.

DNA makes all the basic units of hereditary material which control cellular structure and direct cellular activities. The capacity of the DNA to replicate itself provides the basis of hereditary transmission.

The double helix of DNA

The double helix is made up of two strands of DNA. They twist round each other to resemble a spiral ladder (Figure 1.1). Two strands of alternating phosphate groups and deoxyribose sugars form the uprights of spiral ladder and the paired bases held together by hydrogen bonds form the rungs of the ladder.

RNA

RNA differs from DNA. In humans, RNA is single-stranded (Figure 1.2), the sugar is the pentose sugar and contains the pyrimidine base uracil (U) instead of thymine. Cells have three different RNAs; messenger RNA (mRNA), ribosomal RNA (rRNA) and transfer RNA (tRNA).

Nucleotides

Nucleotides are biological molecules that form the building blocks of nucleic acids (DNA and RNA). A nucleic acid is a chain of repeating monomers called nucleotides. Each nucleotide of DNA consists of three parts (Figure 1.3):

1 Deoxyribose – five-carbon cyclic sugar.
2 Phosphate – an inorganic molecule.
3 Base – a nitro-carbon ring structure.

Bases

Bases are the building blocks of the DNA double helix, and contribute to the folded structure of both DNA and RNA. There are four bases in DNA and these are adenine, thymine, guanine and cytosine. Each base will pair with a particular base as adenine always pairs with thymine and guanine always pairs with cytosine.

Chromosomes

Chromosomes are thread-like structures of DNA found inside a nucleus of a cell (Figure 1.4). Chromosomes also contain DNA-bound proteins, which serve to package the DNA and control its functions. The unique structure of chromosomes keeps DNA tightly wrapped around spool-like proteins, called histones. Without such packaging, DNA molecules would be too long to fit inside cells. Human body cells have 46 chromosomes, 23 inherited from each parent. Each chromosome is a long molecule of DNA.

Protein synthesis

All the genetic information for manufacturing proteins is found in DNA. However, in order to manufacture these proteins, the genetic information encoded in the DNA has to be translated.

In order for this to happen, first the information needs to be transcribed (copied) to produce a specific molecule of RNA. Then the RNA attaches to a ribosome where the information contained in the RNA is translated into a corresponding sequence of amino acids to form a new protein molecule.

Transcription

In transcription, the genetic information contained in the DNA is transcribed into the RNA. Thus the information in the DNA serves as a template for copying the information into a complementary sequence of codons. To do this, the two strands of the DNA are separated and the bases that are attached to each strand then pair up with bases that are attached to the strands of the RNA (Figure 1.5). Transcription of the DNA ends at another special nucleotide sequence called a terminator, which specifies the end of the gene.

Translation

Once mRNA has copied the genetic information from the DNA and is ready for translation, it binds to a specific site on a ribosome. Ribosomes consist of two parts, a large subunit and a small subunit. They contain a binding site for mRNA and two binding sites for tRNA located in the large ribosomal subunit, a P site and a A site. The process of translation occurs as each ribosomes move along the mRNA stand and a new protein is formed.

Gene transference

The process of gene transference can be divided into two stages: mitosis and meiosis.

Mitosis

Mitosis describes the process by which the nucleus of a cell divides to create two new nuclei, each containing an identical copy of DNA. Mitosis can be divided into four stages: prophase, metaphase, anaphase and telophase. Before and after the cells have divided, they enter a stage called interphase. The interphase is often thought to be the resting period of a cell but the cell is busy getting ready for replication.

Meiosis

Meiosis is the process by which certain sex cells are created. The spermatozoa of the male and the ova of the female go through the process of meiosis. Meiosis can be divided into meiosis I and meiosis II. During the interphase that precedes meiosis I, the chromosome of the diploid starts to replicate. As a result each chromosome consists of two identical daughter chromatids. In meiosis II both of the cells produced in meiosis I further divide again.

Meiosis I can be further subdivided into four stages:
• Prophase I
• Metaphase I
• Anaphase I
• Telophase I.
Meiosis II has also four stages:
• Prophase II
• Metaphase II
• Anaphase II
• Telophase II.

2 Homeostatic mechanisms

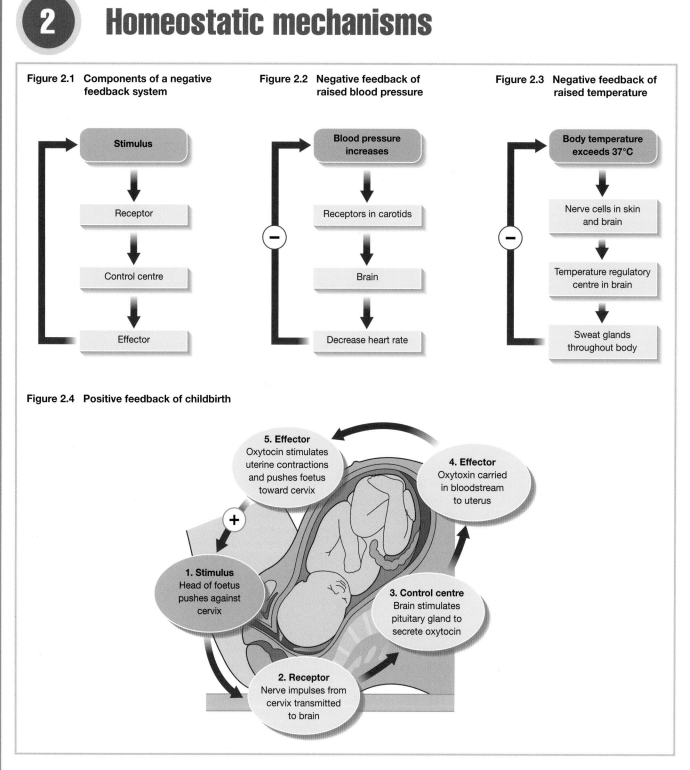

Figure 2.1 Components of a negative feedback system

Stimulus → Receptor → Control centre → Effector

Figure 2.2 Negative feedback of raised blood pressure

Blood pressure increases → Receptors in carotids → Brain → Decrease heart rate
(−)

Figure 2.3 Negative feedback of raised temperature

Body temperature exceeds 37°C → Nerve cells in skin and brain → Temperature regulatory centre in brain → Sweat glands throughout body
(−)

Figure 2.4 Positive feedback of childbirth

5. Effector
Oxytocin stimulates uterine contractions and pushes foetus toward cervix

4. Effector
Oxytoxin carried in bloodstream to uterus

1. Stimulus
Head of foetus pushes against cervix

3. Control centre
Brain stimulates pituitary gland to secrete oxytocin

2. Receptor
Nerve impulses from cervix transmitted to brain

(+)

Homeostasis

Homeostasis is the ability of the body or a cell to seek and maintain a condition of equilibrium within its internal environment when dealing with external changes. It is a state of equilibrium for the body. Homeostasis allows the organs of the body to function effectively in a broad range of conditions. It is an important physiological concept in humans. It was defined by Claude Bernard and later by Walter Bradford Cannon in 1926.

The internal environment includes the tissue fluid that bathes the cells; homeostasis involves keeping various cell conditions within normal limits. Characteristics that are controlled include:

- Temperature – at 36.5°C
- Blood glucose – 4–8 mmol/l
- pH of the blood – at 7.4.

Feedback mechanisms

Our body regulates the internal system through a multitude of feedback systems. There are three basic parts to the feedback system; a receptor, a control centre and an effector (Figure 2.1). The effector can be a muscle, organs or other structure that receives the messages that a reaction is needed.

Receptor

The receptor senses changes in the internal environment and relays information to the control centre. For example certain nerve endings in the skin sense temperature change and detect changes such as a sudden rise or drop in body temperature.

Control centre

The brain is the control centre. It receives the information from the receptor and interprets the information and sends information to the effector. The output could occur as nerve impulses or hormones or other chemical signals.

Effector

An effector is a body system such as the skin, blood vessels or the blood that receives the information from the control centre and produces a response to the condition. For example, the regulation of body temperature by our skin (drops well below normal) where the hypothalamus act as the control centre, which receives input from the skin. The output from the control centre goes to the skeletal muscles via nerves to initiate shivering thus raising body temperature.

Negative feedback

Most of our body systems work on negative feedback. Negative feedback ensures that, in any control system, changes are reversed and returned back to the set level. For example if the right blood pressure increases, receptors in the carotid arteries detect the change in blood pressure and send a message to the brain. The brain will cause the heart to beat slower and thus decrease the blood pressure. Decreasing heart rate has a negative effect on blood pressure (Figure 2.2).

Another example of negative feedback is regulation of our body temperature at a constant 37°C. If we get too hot, blood vessels in our skin vasodilate and we lose heat and cool down. If we get too cold, blood vessels in our skin vasoconstrict, we lose less heat and our body warms up. Thus the negative feedback system ensures the homeostasis is maintained (Figure 2.3).

What happens when the body is too hot?

When the body is too hot the blood vessels (capillaries) in the skin dilate (vasodilation occurs). This activity increases blood to flow to the skin and as this occurs heat is lost through the skin by the processes of convection and radiation. The hairs of the body lie flat (pilorelaxation); this avoids the trapping of air that would otherwise lead to insulation.

Other mechanisms also occur in attempting to further reduce the body temperature, such as sweating. Sweat is produced by the sweat glands and is made up of mostly water and salts and it pours out onto the surface of the skin during increases in temperature. When this occurs the water evaporates, resulting in removal of heat from the skin thus cooling the skin down.

What happens when the body is too cold?

If the body is too cold then hairs on the skin are raised as a result of small muscles making a response, they trap a layer of air near the skin, this gives the appearance of goose bumps (piloerection). When the skeletal muscles contract rapidly and involuntarily shivering occurs. In turn this produces more heat, and during shivering there is often an increase in the rate of respiration, which also helps to warm the surrounding tissues.

The rate at which heat is lost will depend on the amount of blood that is flowing through the skin. When cold, blood is kept away from the body surface as a result of capillary vasoconstriction (reduction in the size of the vessels), smaller amounts of blood flow through these capillaries minimising heat loss from the skin.

Positive feedback

Positive feedback is the body's mechanism to enhance an output needed to maintain homeostasis. Positive feedback mechanisms push levels out of normal ranges. Even though this process can be beneficial, it is rarely used by the body because of the risk of the increased stimuli becoming out of control. An example of positive feedback is the release of oxytocin to increase and keep the contractions of childbirth happening as long as needed for the child's birth. Contractions of the uterus are stimulated by oxytocin, produced in the pituitary gland, and the secretion of it is increased by positive feedback, increasing the strength of the contractions (Figure 2.4).

3 Fluid compartments

Figure 3.1 Distribution of body water

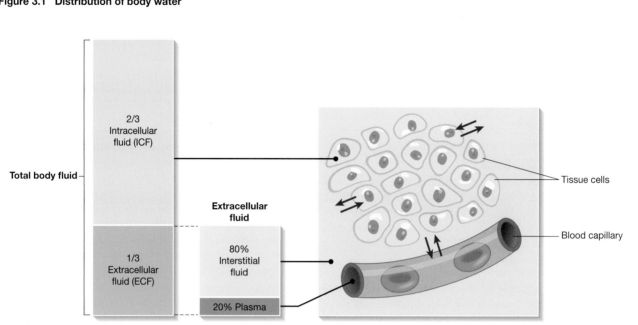

Source: Nair, M & Peate I Fundamentals of Applied Pathophysiology (2013)

Table 3.1 Fluid intake and losses

Fluid source			Fluid loss	
Oral liquids	1200 – 1500 ml daily		Urine	1200 – 1700 ml daily
Food	700 – 1000 ml daily		Faeces	100 – 250 ml daily
Metabolism	200 – 400 ml daily		Perspiration	100 – 150 ml daily
			Insensible loss	
			Skin	350 – 400 ml daily
			Lungs	350 – 400 ml daily
Total	**2100 – 2900 ml daily**		**Total**	**2100 – 2900 ml daily**
Average intake	2500 ml daily		Average loss	2500 ml daily

Water is the universal solvent and is essential for life, and body fluids are dilute solutions of water and electrolytes. It is an extraordinary substance with a number of important properties.

Total body water

It is estimated that the total body water in an adult of average build amounts to about 60% of their body weight. There are, however, some exceptions to this; for example, in babies and young people the proportion will be higher, conversely, in those adults who are below average weight, the proportion will be lower, this also applies to the elderly and to the obese in all age groups. Total body water therefore depends upon a number of factors that include sex, weight, age and relative amount of body fat, as we age total body water declines and as such the risk of experiencing a fluid imbalance increases with age.

The difference between males and females is due to the fact that women have a relatively larger amount of body fat as well as a smaller amount of skeletal muscle. Skeletal muscle is composed of 65% water; adipose tissue, however, is only about 20% water. Those people with a greater muscle mass have proportionately more body water, an obese person can have a relative water content level as low as 45%.

There are two major biochemically distinct fluid compartments in the body where body fluids are distributed; inside the cells (intracellular) and outside the cells (extracellular).

Figure 3.1 provides details about the distribution of body water.

Blood is a life maintaining fluid and is the only liquid connective tissue, comprising 8% of total body weight (and consists of red blood cells (erythrocytes), plasma, white blood cells (leukocytes) and platelets (thrombocytes). One key aspect related to the role of the blood is to help transport gases, nutrients and waste products, provide a defence against infection and injury, assist in the immune process and contribute to the regulation of temperature, acid base balance and fluid exchange.

In order for cells to function effectively this depends on a stable supply of nutrients, the removal of waste products and also on homeostasis of the surrounding fluids. Fluctuations in fluids impacts upon blood volume and cellular function, alterations in cellular function can be life threatening.

Intracellular fluid

In an adult nearly two thirds of the body's fluid is intracellular (ICF) and this is contained within more than 100 trillion cells, amounting to approximately 28 litres an average 70 kg male. These vast numbers of cells are not united physically; the intracellular fluid compartment is in fact a virtual compartment. These are discontinuous small collections of fluid; however, from a physiological perspective, intracellular fluid is discussed as if it were a single compartment.

Extracellular fluid

Extracellular fluid (ECF) is the fluid that is found outside of cells but surrounding them. ECF also declines as we age, ECF is more readily lost from the body than the ICF. ECF is usually subdivided into a number of smaller compartments located in the intravascular and the interstitial compartments or spaces. The intravascular compartment consists of fluid within the blood vessels (the plasma volume). In an average adult blood volume amounts to 5–6 litres, of this approximately 3 litres is plasma. The interstitial fluid is water in the 'gaps' between the cells and outside the blood vessels this also includes lymph fluid (sometimes this is called the 'third space'). Transcellular fluid is fluid that is contained within particular cavities of the body, for example, the pleural, synovial, pericardial fluids and digestive secretions that are separated by a layer of epithelium from the interstitial compartment. Transcellular fluid is akin to interstitial fluid and often this is considered to be a part of interstitial volume. The transcellular fluid amounts to about 1 litre.

The plasma membrane

The plasma membrane divides the intracellular and extracellular compartments and specialised cell layers divide the interstitial and transcellular compartments. The capillary wall divides the blood from the interstitial fluid. The capillary wall is a semipermeable membrane; this is permeable to most molecules in the plasma except plasma proteins and the red blood cells as these are too large to move through the capillary wall. This selective permeability assists in maintaining the unique composition of the compartments and at the same time allowing the transportation of nutrients from the plasma to the cells and the passage of waste products from the cells out into the plasma.

Fluid regulation

There is a fine regulation of the balance between water intake and output and its distribution is essential to the optimal performance of every organ system in the body. In a number of illnesses and during surgery, there may be disturbances that occur to this fine balance, this must be identified and corrected with the aim of preventing deterioration, complications and to promote recovery.

In adults who are healthy, fluid intake usually averages about 2200 ml per day, this can range from 1800 ml per day with similar fluid loss (see Table 3.1). In normal circumstances there are a number of bodily mechanisms that ensure that there is a state of equilibrium between intake and output. The brain triggers the sensation of thirst when body fluid becomes concentrated, this then encourages the person to drink. When fluid volume expands then the kidneys will excrete a proportionate amount of water to correct, maintain or restore balance.

4 Cells and organelles

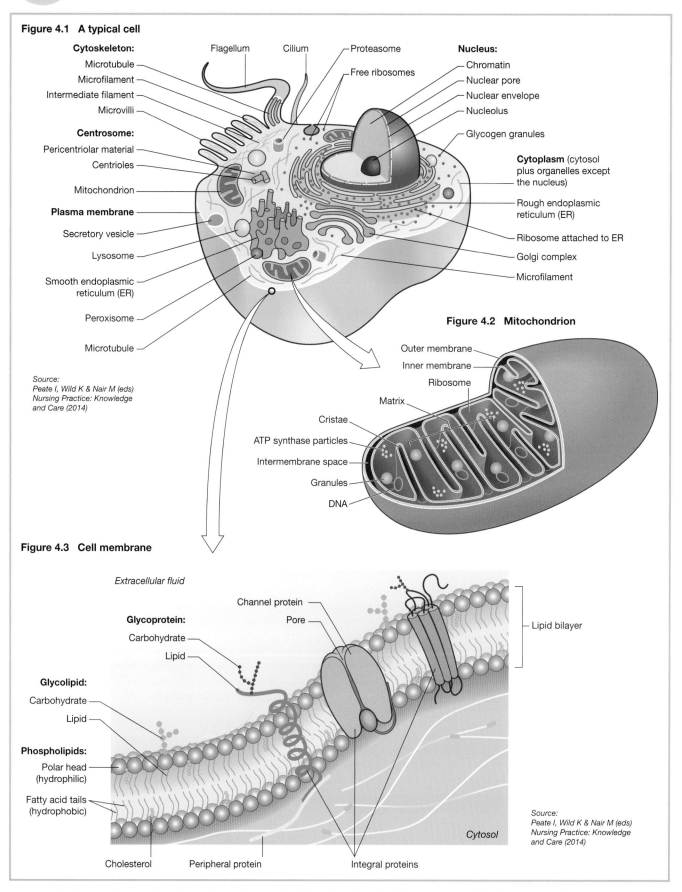

Figure 4.1   A typical cell

Cytoskeleton:
Microtubule
Microfilament
Intermediate filament
Microvilli

Centrosome:
Pericentriolar material
Centrioles

Mitochondrion

Plasma membrane

Secretory vesicle

Lysosome

Smooth endoplasmic reticulum (ER)

Peroxisome

Microtubule

Flagellum

Cilium

Proteasome

Free ribosomes

Nucleus:
Chromatin
Nuclear pore
Nuclear envelope
Nucleolus

Glycogen granules

Cytoplasm (cytosol plus organelles except the nucleus)

Rough endoplasmic reticulum (ER)

Ribosome attached to ER

Golgi complex

Microfilament

Source:
Peate I, Wild K & Nair M (eds)
Nursing Practice: Knowledge and Care (2014)

Figure 4.2   Mitochondrion

Outer membrane
Inner membrane
Ribosome
Matrix
Cristae
ATP synthase particles
Intermembrane space
Granules
DNA

Figure 4.3   Cell membrane

Extracellular fluid

Channel protein
Pore

Glycoprotein:
Carbohydrate
Lipid

Lipid bilayer

Glycolipid:
Carbohydrate
Lipid

Phospholipids:
Polar head (hydrophilic)
Fatty acid tails (hydrophobic)

Cytosol

Source:
Peate I, Wild K & Nair M (eds)
Nursing Practice: Knowledge and Care (2014)

Cholesterol   Peripheral protein   Integral proteins

Anatomy and Physiology for Nurses at a Glance, First Edition. Ian Peate and Muralitharan Nair. © 2015 John Wiley & Sons, Ltd. Published 2015 by John Wiley & Sons, Ltd.
Companion website: www.ataglanceseries.com/nursing/anatomy

Cells

Cells are the basic structural, functional and biological unit of all known living organisms. We humans are multicellular, compared to some organisms such as bacteria. Each cell is an amazing world unto itself: it can take in nutrients, convert these nutrients into energy, carry out specialised functions, and reproduce as necessary.

Cell membrane

This membrane serves to separate and protect a cell from its surrounding environment and is made mostly from a double layer of proteins and lipids, fat-like molecules. Embedded within this membrane are a variety of other molecules (Figure 4.1) that act as channels and pumps, moving different molecules into and out of the cell. The cell membrane can vary from 7.5 nanometres (nm) to 10 nm in thickness.

The phospholipid bilayer consists of a polar 'head' end which is hydrophilic (water loving) and fatty acid 'tails' which are hydrophobic (water hating). The hydrophilic heads are situated on the outer and inner surface of the cell while the hydrophobic areas point into the cell membrane (see Figure 4.1) as they are 'water hating' ends. These phospholipid molecules are arranged as a bilayer with the heads facing outwards. This means that the bilayer is self-sealing. It is the central part of the cell membrane, consisting of hydrophobic 'tails', that makes the cell membrane impermeable to water-soluble molecules, and so prevents the passage of these molecules into and out of the cell.

Mitochondria

Mitochondria (Figure 4.2) are the cell's power producers. They convert energy into forms that are usable by the cell. Located in the cytoplasm, they are the sites of cellular respiration which ultimately generate fuel for the cell's activities. Mitochondria are also involved in other cell processes, such as cell division and growth, as well as cell death.

Endoplasmic reticulum

The endoplasmic reticulum (ER) (Figure 4.1) is an organelle of cells that forms an interconnected network of membrane vesicles. According to the structure, the endoplasmic reticulum is classified into two types, that is, rough endoplasmic reticulum (RER) and smooth endoplasmic reticulum (SER). The rough endoplasmic reticulum is studded with ribosomes on the cytosolic face. These are the sites of protein synthesis. The rough endoplasmic reticulum is predominantly found in hepatocytes where protein synthesis occurs actively. The smooth endoplasmic reticulum is a smooth network without the ribosomes. The smooth endoplasmic reticulum is concerned with lipid metabolism, carbohydrate metabolism and detoxification. The smooth endoplasmic reticulum is abundantly found in mammalian liver and gonad cells.

Nucleus

The nucleus is a membrane-enclosed organelle (Figure 4.1). It contains most of the cell's genetic material, organised as multiple long linear DNA molecules in complex with a large variety of proteins, such as histones, to form chromosomes. The genes within these chromosomes are the cell's nuclear genome. The function of the nucleus is to maintain the integrity of these genes and to control the activities of the cell by regulating gene expression — the nucleus is, therefore, the control centre of the cell.

Cytoplasm

Cytoplasm is basically the substance that fills the cell. It is a jelly-like material that is 80% water and is usually clear in colour. It is more like a viscous (thick) gel than a watery substance, but it liquefies when shaken or stirred. Cytoplasm, which can also be referred to as cytosol, means cell substance. This name is very fitting because cytoplasm is the substance of life that serves as a molecular soup in which all of the cell's organelles are suspended and held together by a fatty membrane. The cytoplasm is found inside the cell membrane, surrounding the nuclear envelope and the cytoplasmic organelles (Figure 4.1).

Lipid bilayer

The lipid bilayer is a thin polar membrane made of two layers of lipid molecules that keeps ions, proteins and other molecules where they are needed and prevents them from diffusing into areas where they should not be. The lipid layer is made up of three types of lipid molecules: phospholipids (75%), cholesterol (20%) and glycolipids (5%).

The polar heads are hydrophilic (water loving) and in contact with both the extracellular fluid and the cytosol. While the fatty acid tails, which are hydrophobic (water fearing), point towards each other inside the membrane (Figure 4.3).

Membrane proteins

Membrane proteins are categorised as integral or peripheral proteins (Figure 4.3). Integral proteins extend through the lipid layer into the cytosol of the cell. Thus some of the small molecules can pass from the extracellular fluid through to the intracellular fluid.

Peripheral proteins do not go through the lipid layer. They are more associated with the polar heads of both outer and inner surfaces of the membrane.

Functions of the plasma membrane

The cell membrane anchors the cytoskeleton (a cellular 'skeleton' made of protein and contained in the cytoplasm) and gives shape to the cell.

It attaches cells to the extracellular matrix and transports materials in and out of the cells. Some protein molecules in the cell membrane carry out metabolic reactions near the inner surface of the cell membrane.

5 Transport systems

Figure 5.1 Osmosis

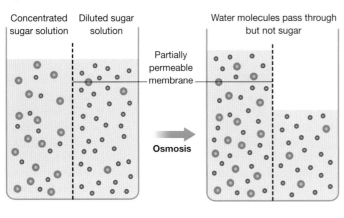

Concentrated sugar solution | Diluted sugar solution | Water molecules pass through but not sugar

Partially permeable membrane

Osmosis

- ◉ Sugar molecules
- ● Water molecules

Figure 5.2 Simple diffusion

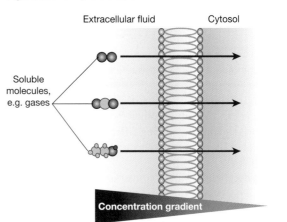

Extracellular fluid | Cytosol

Soluble molecules, e.g. gases

Concentration gradient

Source: Peate I, Wild K & Nair M (eds) Nursing Practice: Knowledge and Care (2014)

Figure 5.3 Active transport

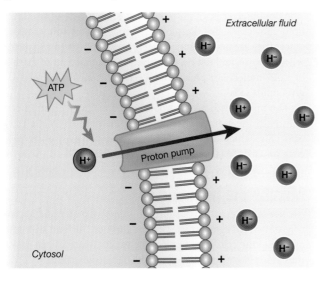

Extracellular fluid

ATP

Proton pump

H+

Cytosol

Figure 5.4 Facilitated diffusion

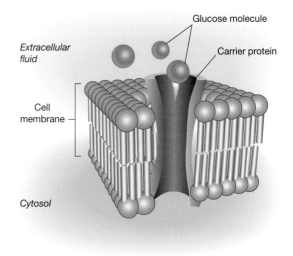

Glucose molecule

Carrier protein

Extracellular fluid

Cell membrane

Cytosol

Source: Peate I, Wild K & Nair M (eds) Nursing Practice: Knowledge and Care (2014)

Figure 5.5 Endocytosis

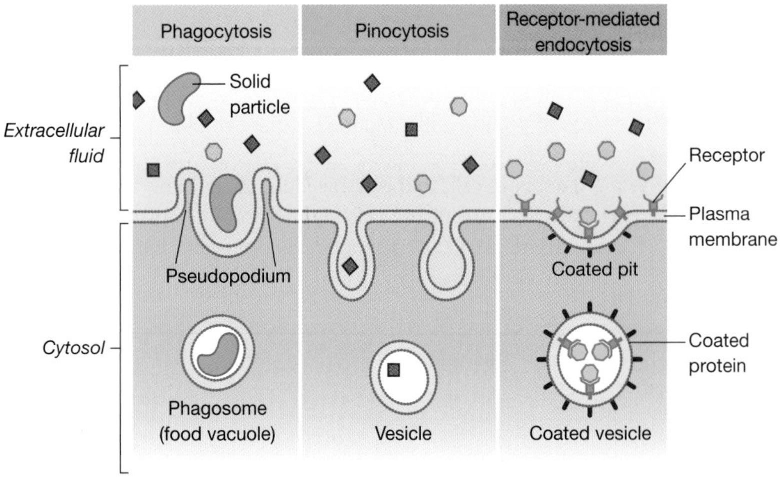

Phagocytosis | Pinocytosis | Receptor-mediated endocytosis

Extracellular fluid

Solid particle

Cytosol

Pseudopodium

Phagosome (food vacuole)

Vesicle

Receptor

Plasma membrane

Coated pit

Coated protein

Coated vesicle

Figure 5.6 Exocytosis

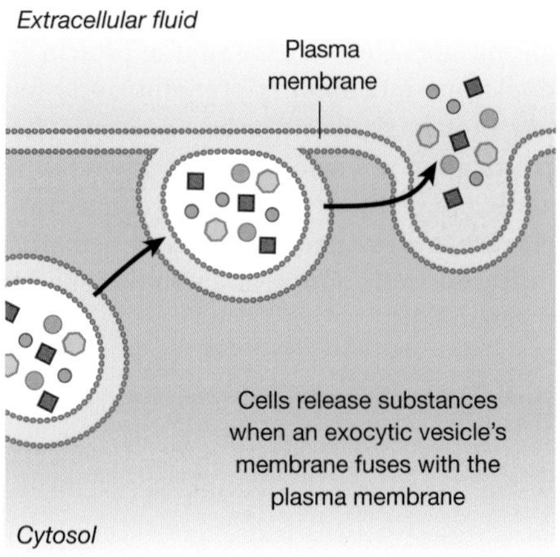

Extracellular fluid

Plasma membrane

Cells release substances when an exocytic vesicle's membrane fuses with the plasma membrane

Cytosol

Anatomy and Physiology for Nurses at a Glance, First Edition. Ian Peate and Muralitharan Nair. © 2015 John Wiley & Sons, Ltd. Published 2015 by John Wiley & Sons, Ltd.
Companion website: www.ataglanceseries.com/nursing/anatomy

Osmosis

Osmosis is the movement of solution from an area of high volume to an area of low volume through a selective permeable membrane. Osmosis is essential in biological systems, as biological membranes are selective permeable (Figure 5.1). Although osmosis does not utilise energy, it does use kinetic energy. The kinetic energy of an object is the energy which it possesses due to its movement. The movement of water driven by osmosis is called osmotic flow. The greater the initial difference in solute concentrations, the stronger the osmotic flow.

Solutions of varying solute concentration are described as isotonic, hypotonic or hypertonic. When a cell is placed in an isotonic solution there is very little net movement of water in or out of the cell. When placed in a hypotonic solution water will move into the cell causing it to swell and burst. However, when the cell is placed in a hypertonic solution, the water will move out of the cell causing to shrink and die.

Diffusion

Diffusion is the net movement of molecules from an area of high concentration to an area of low concentration. The difference between the high and low concentration represents the concentration gradient. Diffusion occurs in air as well as in water. Although the process is spontaneous, the rate of diffusion for different substances is affected by membrane permeability. The rate of diffusion is also affected by properties of the cell, the diffusing molecule, temperature of the surrounding solution and the size of the molecule.

Simple passive diffusion occurs when small molecules pass through the lipid bilayer of a cell membrane, for example gas exchange in the lungs (Figure 5.2).

Facilitated diffusion

Facilitated diffusion is a type of passive transport that allows substances to cross membranes with the assistance of special transport proteins (Figure 5.4). The facilitated diffusion may occur either across biological membranes or through fluid compartments. The molecule to be transported first binds to a receptor site on the carrier protein. The shape of the protein then changes and the molecule is transported into the cell where it is released into the cytoplasm. Once the transport is complete, the protein returns to its normal shape.

Active transport

In active transport, the high energy bond in ATP (adeinosinetriphosphate) provides the energy needed to move ions or molecules across the membrane (Figure 5.3). Active transport is not dependent on the concentration gradient. As a result, cells can take in or get rid of molecules regardless of the concentration of the molecules in the intracellular or the extracellular fluid

compartments. It is a good example of a process for which cells require energy. Examples of active transport include the uptake of glucose in the intestines. All cells contain carrier proteins called ion pumps, which actively transport ions such as sodium or potassium across the cell membranes.

Secondary active transport

Secondary active transport is a form of active transport across a biological membrane in which a transporter protein couples the movement of an ion (typically Na^+ or H^+) down its electrochemical gradient to the uphill movement of another molecule or ion against a concentration/electrochemical gradient. In secondary active transport, the free energy needed to perform active transport is provided by the concentration gradient of the driving ion.

Endocytosis and exocytosis

Endocytosis is an energy-using process by which cells absorb molecules (such as proteins) by engulfing them. Endocytosis (Figure 5.5) occurs in three different ways:

i Phagocytosis: Pseudopodia engulf the particle to be imported to create a food vacuole. Once inside the cell, a lysosyme containing digestive enzymes will fuse with the food vacuole.

ii Pinocytosis: The cell membrane pinches in to engulf a portion of extracellular fluid containing solutes required by the cell. This process is non-specific; any solutes in the solution will be engulfed.

iii Receptor-mediated endocytosis: This process allows the intake of large quantities of molecules that may not be in high concentration in the extracellular fluid. Proteins on the surface have specific receptor sites that bind to specific molecules. Receptors then cluster in coated pits, which are covered on the cytoplasm side with coat proteins. The coated pit pinches off as a vesicle, taking with it high concentrations of the specified molecule but also some other molecules from the extracellular fluid. After the molecules are delivered to their destination, the receptor proteins are recycled to the plasma membrane.

Exocytosis is the process in which the cell releases materials to the outside by discharging them as membrane-bounded vesicles passing through the cell membrane (Figure 5.6). Exocytosis can be constitutive (occurring all the time) or regulated.

Purpose of exocytosis

Many cells in the body use exocytosis to release enzymes or other proteins that act in other areas of the body or to release molecules that help cells communicate with one another. For instance, clusters of α- and β-cells in the islets of Langerhans in the pancreas secrete the hormones glucagon and insulin, respectively. These enzymes regulate glucose levels throughout the body. As the level of glucose rises in the blood, the β-cells are stimulated to produce and secrete more insulin by exocytosis. When insulin binds to liver or muscle, it stimulates uptake of glucose by those cells. Exocytosis from other cells in the pancreas also releases digestive enzymes into the gut.

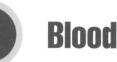 **Blood**

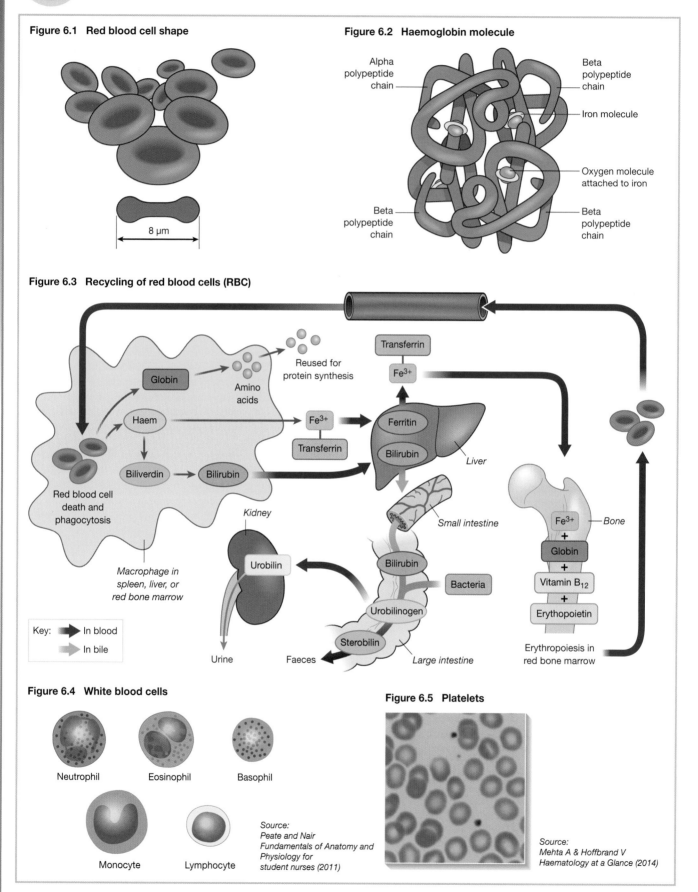

Figure 6.1 Red blood cell shape

8 µm

Figure 6.2 Haemoglobin molecule

Alpha polypeptide chain

Beta polypeptide chain

Iron molecule

Oxygen molecule attached to iron

Beta polypeptide chain

Beta polypeptide chain

Figure 6.3 Recycling of red blood cells (RBC)

Globin

Amino acids

Reused for protein synthesis

Transferrin

Fe^{3+}

Haem

Fe^{3+}

Transferrin

Ferritin

Bilirubin

Liver

Biliverdin

Bilirubin

Red blood cell death and phagocytosis

Macrophage in spleen, liver, or red bone marrow

Kidney

Urobilin

Small intestine

Bilirubin

Bacteria

Urobilinogen

Sterobilin

Urine

Faeces

Large intestine

Bone

Fe^{3+}
+
Globin
+
Vitamin B_{12}
+
Erythopoietin

Erythropoiesis in red bone marrow

Key:
➤ In blood
➤ In bile

Figure 6.4 White blood cells

Neutrophil

Eosinophil

Basophil

Monocyte

Lymphocyte

*Source:
Peate and Nair
Fundamentals of Anatomy and
Physiology for
student nurses (2011)*

Figure 6.5 Platelets

*Source:
Mehta A & Hoffbrand V
Haematology at a Glance (2014)*

Anatomy and Physiology for Nurses at a Glance, First Edition. Ian Peate and Muralitharan Nair. © 2015 John Wiley & Sons, Ltd. Published 2015 by John Wiley & Sons, Ltd.
Companion website: www.ataglanceseries.com/nursing/anatomy

Blood

Blood is a fluid connective tissue. Blood consists of formed elements such red blood cells (RBC), white blood cells (WBC), platelets and a fluid portion called plasma. The volume of blood between men and women differs as a result of body size. Adult men have approximately 5–6 litres and adult women have 4–5 litres of blood.

Formation of blood cells

The process by which formed elements of blood develop is called haemopoiesis. Red bone marrow is the primary centre for haemopoiesis in the last three months of birth and throughout life.

RBC

RBCs also known as erythrocytes are the most abundant blood cells. They are biconcave disks (Figure 6.1) and they contain oxygen-carrying protein called haemoglobin. The biconcave shape is maintained by a network of proteins called spectrin. This network of protein will allow the red blood cells to change shape as they are transported through the blood vessel. Young red blood cells contain a nucleus; however, the nucleus is absent in a mature red blood cell which is without any organelles such as mitochondria thus increasing the oxygen carrying capacity of the red blood cell.

Haemoglobin

Haemoglobin is composed of the protein called globin bound to the iron containing pigments called haem. Each globin molecule has four polypeptide chains consisting of 2 alpha and 2 beta chains (Figure 6.2). Each haemoglobin molecule has 4 atoms of iron and each atom of iron will transport 1 molecule of oxygen, therefore, 1 molecule of haemoglobin will transport 4 molecules of oxygen. There are approximately 250 million haemoglobin molecules in one red blood cell and therefore one red blood cell will transport 1 billion molecules of oxygen.

Recycling of RBC

Without a nucleus and other organelles the red blood cell cannot synthesise new structures to replace the ones that are damaged and therefore their life span is approximately 3–4 months. The breakdown (haemolysis) of the red blood cell is carried out by macrophages in the spleen, liver and the bone marrow (Figure 6.3). The globin is broken down and reused for protein synthesis. Iron is removed and stored in the muscles and the liver and reused to manufacture new red blood cells.

WBC

WBC circulates for only a short portion of their life span. They spend most of their life span migrating through dense and loose connective tissues throughout the body. All white blood cells migrate from the blood vessel by a process called emigration. Some of the white blood cells are capable of phagocytosis and they are neutrophils, eosinophils and monocytes.

Neutrophils

Neotrophils are the most abundant white blood cells and play an important role in the immune system. They form approximately 60–65% of granulocytes and are phagocytes. A non-active neutrophil lasts approximately 12 hours while an active neutrophil could last 1–2 days. Neutrophils are the first immune cells to arrive at a site of infection, through a process known as chemotaxis. The nuclei of the neutrophils are multi-lobed (Figure 6.4).

Eosinophils

These form approximately 2–4% of granulocytes and have B-shaped nuclei (Figure 6.4). Like neutrophils, they too migrate from blood vessels and they are 10–12 μm in diameter. They are phagocytes; however, they are not as active as neutrophils. They contain lysosomal enzymes and peroxidase in their granules, which is toxic to parasites resulting in the destruction of the organism.

Basophil

Basophils are the least abundant and account for approximately 1% of granulocytes, they contain elongated lobed nuclei (Figure 6.4). Basophils are 8–10 μm in diameter. In inflamed tissue they become mast cells and secrete granules containing heparin, histamine and other proteins that promote inflammation.

Monocytes

Monocytes account for 5% of the agranulocytes and they are circulating leucocytes (Figure 6.4). Monocytes develop in the bone marrow and spread through the body in 1–3 days. They are approximately 12–20 μm in diameter. The nucleus of the monocyte is kidney or horseshoe shaped. Macrophages play a vital role in immunity and inflammation by destroying specific antigens.

Lymphocytes

Lymphocytes account for 25% of the leucocytes and most are found in the lymphatic tissue such as the lymph nodes and the spleen (see Figure 6.4). Small lymphocytes are approximately 6–9 μm in diameter while the larger ones are 10–14 μm in diameter. They can leave and re-enter the circulatory system. The life span of the lymphocytes ranges from a few hours to years.

Platelets

Platelets are small blood cells consisting of some cytoplasm surrounded by a plasma membrane. They are produced in the bone marrow from megakaryocytes (Figure 6.5) and fragments of megakaryocytes break off to form platelets. They are approximately 2–4 μm in diameter but have no nucleus and their life span is approximately 5–9 days. Platelets play a vital role in blood loss by the formation of platelet plugs which seal the holes in the blood vessels and release chemicals which aid blood clotting.

Blood plasma

Blood plasma is a pale yellow coloured fluid and its total volume is approximately 2.5–3 litres in adults. Plasma is 91% water and 10% solutes such electrolytes and plasma proteins. Among other roles, blood plasma proteins maintain blood osmotic pressure, which is an important factor in fluid exchange.

7 Inflammation and immunity

Figure 7.1 The cells of the immune system

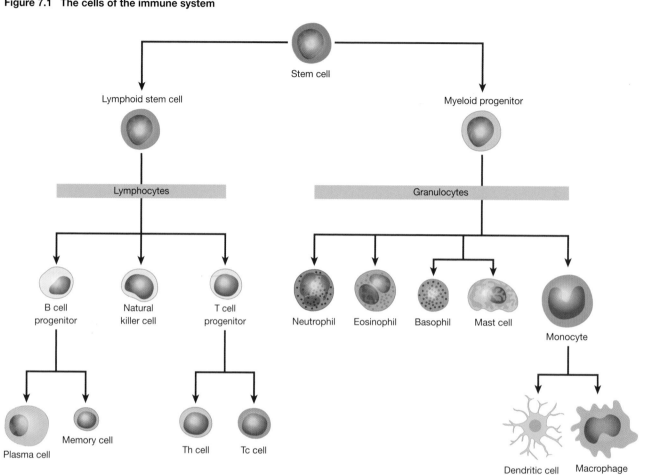

Stem cell

Lymphoid stem cell

Myeloid progenitor

Lymphocytes

Granulocytes

B cell progenitor

Natural killer cell

T cell progenitor

Neutrophil Eosinophil Basophil Mast cell

Monocyte

Plasma cell Memory cell

Th cell Tc cell

Dendritic cell Macrophage

Table 7.1 Types of antibodies

Type of antibody	Functions
IgA	Found in breast milk, mucous, saliva and tears prevents antigens from crossing epithelial membranes and invading the deeper tissues
IgD	Produced by B cells and is displayed on their surface. Antigens bind to active B cells here
IgE	The last common antibody. Found bound to tissue cell membranes particularly eosinophils
IgG	The most common and largest antibody. Attacks various pathogens, crossing the placenta to protect the foetus
IgM	Produced in large quantities, is the primary response and a powerful activator of complement

Figure 7.2 Types of acquired immunity

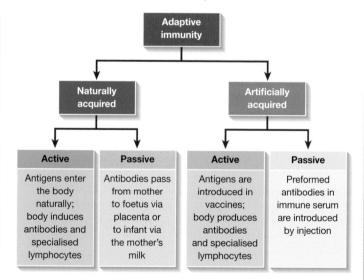

	Active	Passive	Active	Passive
Adaptive immunity				
Naturally acquired	Antigens enter the body naturally; body induces antibodies and specialised lymphocytes	Antibodies pass from mother to foetus via placenta or to infant via the mother's milk		
Artificially acquired			Antigens are introduced in vaccines; body produces antibodies and specialised lymphocytes	Preformed antibodies in immune serum are introduced by injection

Haemostasis and haemostatic mechanisms are responsible for the clotting of blood once injury or damage occurs to the skin. This happens through a number of complex mechanisms that culminate in the production of a blood clot and scab formation, providing protection as damage to the external surfaces of the body can allow routes of entry for foreign bodies as well as pathogenic microorganisms.

Immune system

Throughout our lives we depend on the immune system to protect us from the moment we are born until we die. Almost every disease, accident or disorder we have has an association with the immune system. The immune system is concerned with more than infections.

The body is constantly exposed to a number of foreign substances, infectious agents as well as abnormal cells, and the immune system is the key defender in protection.

The immune system is an intricate system of cells, enzymes and proteins providing protection and rendering us resistant or immune to infections caused by various microorganisms, for example, bacteria, viruses and fungi. The immune system is capable of doing more than fighting infection and protecting us from infectious diseases, other functions include the removal and destruction of damaged or dead cells and the identification and destruction of malignant cells, helping to prevent them from further development into tumours.

Types of immunity

There are two types of immunity: the innate and the acquired.

Innate immunity

This is acquired at birth. The foetus acquires some immunity via the placenta, this is called passive immunity and lasts for about 3–6 months; the main antibody which is able to cross the placenta is immunoglobulin IgG. Although the time period for providing this passive immunity is limited, it is important at a time when the immune system is immature. After about 6 months infants are more prone to respiratory and gastric infections. This is in part due to the loss of foetal antibodies before the B and T lymphocytes are fully immunocompetent. A central role of the innate immune responses is to prevent or restrict the entrance of microorganisms into the body, so that tissue damage is limited. Inflammation is an example of an innate immune response (also called non-specific immunity).

Inflammation

When tissue damage occurs this activates a number of proteins acting as the catalyst for the immune response. This response is non-specific attacking any and all foreign invaders attempting to rid the body of microbes, toxins or other foreign matter, aiming to prevent their spread to other tissues and prepare the site for tissue repair, restoring tissue homeostasis.

The responsibilities of the cells of the immune system are to find and destroy any damaged cells and foreign tissues and simultaneously recognise and preserve host cells.

There are four phases related to the inflammatory response:

1 redness
2 swelling
3 heat
4 pain.

When injury occurs, almost instantaneously the damaged cells cause a number of events to happen: vasodilation, release of messenger molecules, initiation of complement, extravasation of vascular components, phagocytosis and pain.

The injured mast cells release histamine, causing arterioles to dilate and venules to constrict promoting an increase in blood flow. The main mechanisms associated with vasodilation are: cells produce bradykinin (a vasodilator, also causes pain), damaged plasma membranes release arachidonic acid, a fatty acid, a precursor to prostaglandins. Prostaglandins (vasodilators) can increase pain. The histamine released from the degranulated mast cells enlarges pore size between the capillary cells permitting proteins and other micromolecules to move into the interstitial spaces. Nitric oxide is released by the vascular epithelial cells causing further vasodilation; the presence of macrophages releases large quantities of nitric oxide.

Cells close to the injury release a series of chemical signals radiating from the site of inflammation – chemokines. The concentration of chemokines is greatest immediately surrounding the infection, high levels of chemokines provide a signal for the attraction of phagocytic white blood cells including neutrophils. Figure 7.1 outlines the cells of the immune system.

As chemokine concentration increases, the phagocytes leave the capillary and enter the site of infection, macrophages arrive around 24 hours later. The phagocytes engulf and destroy the pathogens present recognising this as non-self matter. The key molecule released is interleukin 1 attracting neutrophils and macrophages to the site of injury and helping to clear away debris from the injured area.

Acquired immunity

Also known as specific immunity as it only responds to known, specific organisms that we have previously encountered (have previously infected us). Acquired immunity has the ability to remember when a particular immunological threat has been met and overcome, remembering how to defeat it and mobilise the immune system to counter that threat (immunological memory). The acquired immune system is based upon the lymphocytes that are closely associated to the lymphatic system.

The primary response (exposure for the first time) generates a slow and delayed rise in antibody levels. The delay is associated with activation of the T lymphocyte system that stimulates B lymphocyte separation.

The secondary response occurs on subsequent exposure to the same antigen and the response in this case is much faster as the memory B lymphocytes generated after the first infection divide and separate at a much faster rate, antibody production occurs almost immediately. See Table 7.1 for the five types of antibody.

Natural and artificial acquired immunity

Immunity can be acquired naturally or artificially, both forms can be active or passive (see Figure 7.2).

When active immunity occurs, this means that the person has made a response to an antigen and this leads to the production of their own antibodies with activation of the lymphocytes, the memory cells offer long lasting resistance.

Passive immunity occurs when the person has been given antibodies. This type of immunity is relatively short acting as the antibodies eventually break down.

8 Tissues

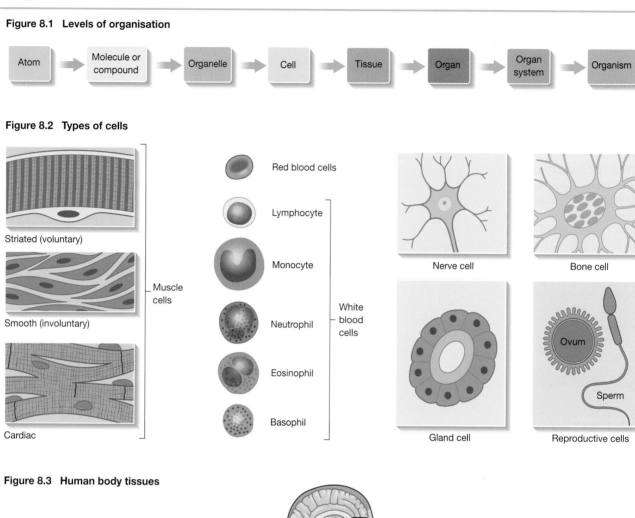

Figure 8.1 Levels of organisation

Atom → Molecule or compound → Organelle → Cell → Tissue → Organ → Organ system → Organism

Figure 8.2 Types of cells

Striated (voluntary)

Smooth (involuntary)

Cardiac

} Muscle cells

Red blood cells

Lymphocyte

Monocyte

Neutrophil

Eosinophil

Basophil

} White blood cells

Nerve cell

Bone cell

Gland cell

Reproductive cells
Ovum
Sperm

Figure 8.3 Human body tissues

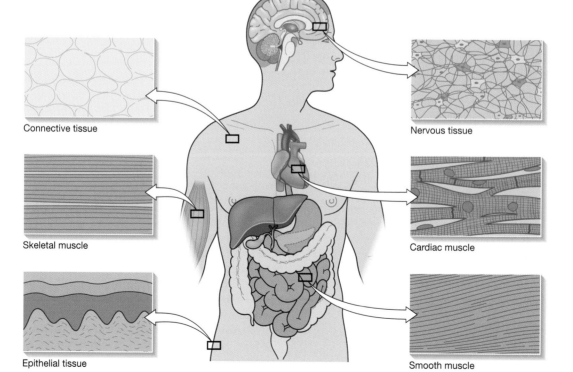

Connective tissue

Nervous tissue

Skeletal muscle

Cardiac muscle

Epithelial tissue

Smooth muscle

Anatomy and Physiology for Nurses at a Glance, First Edition. Ian Peate and Muralitharan Nair. © 2015 John Wiley & Sons, Ltd. Published 2015 by John Wiley & Sons, Ltd.
Companion website: www.ataglanceseries.com/nursing/anatomy

Chapter 4 explained the physiological environment of the cell. The basic building blocks of organisms are the cells. Humans are complex beings and are comprised of many cells, which are different sizes and shapes and have various functions.

Tissues

Tissues are made up of large numbers of cells and are classified according to their size, shape and functions (see Figures 8.1, 8.2, 8.3). With each tissue type there are wide variations in their cellular morphology as well as their function. Generally tissue types are made up of similar cells carrying out related functions, for example, the epidermis of the face and the lining of the mouth are the same tissue type and have related functions, yet their appearance is very different when observed by the naked eye. Blood and bone are the same type of tissue but they look very different. There are four main types of tissues, each has its own sub divisions and they are:

- epithelial tissue
- nervous tissue
- connective tissue
- muscle tissue.

Epithelial tissue

Epithelial tissue, also known as epithelia, is located in the covering of external and internal surfaces of the body, the hollow organs and tubes, it is also found in the glands. The overall function of the epithelium is to provide protection and impermeability (or selective permeability) to the covered structure.

The cells are closely packed and the matrix (the intracellular substance) is minimal. There is usually a basement membrane on which the cells lie. The epithelial tissue may be simple (a single layer of cells) and this is subdivided into squamous epithelium (forms the lining of the heart, blood vessels, lymph vessels, alveoli of the lungs, lining of the collecting ducts of the nephrons) or stratified where there are several layers of tissue and this is composed of several layers of these cells. Keratinised stratified epithelium is found on those dry surfaces that are exposed to wear and tear; for example, the skin, hair and nails. Non-keratinised epithelium protects those moist surfaces that are subjected to wear and tear, this tissue type prevents surfaces such as the conjunctiva, the linings of the mouth and the vagina from drying out. The urinary bladder is lined with transitional epithelium – this permits the bladder to stretch as it fills.

Nervous tissue

Nervous tissue is made up of neurons and glial cells. The function of the nervous tissue is to receive and to transmit neural impulses (reception and transmission of information). There are two types of tissue found in the nervous system: excitable cells (the neurons – they initiate, receive, conduct and transmit information) and the non-excitable cells (the glial cells – these support the neurons).

A neuron (the basic unit of nervous tissue) consists of two major parts, the cell body containing the neuron's nucleus, cytoplasm and other organelles. The nerve processes are 'finger-like' projections arising from the cell body and are able to conduct and transmit signals. There are two types: the axons that carry signals away from the cell body and the dendrites carrying signals toward the cell body. Neurons usually have one axon (this can be branched). Axons usually terminate at a synapse through which the signal is sent to the next cell, usually through a dendrite.

Connective tissue

There are a number of varieties of connective tissue, it is the most abundant type of tissue; the typical function of connective tissue is to fill empty spaces among other body tissues. This function is associated with the ability of the cells of the connective tissue to secrete substances that compose extracellular material, such as collagen and elastic fibres, creating a significant spacing between these cells. There are other important biological features of the connective tissues, including substance transportation, protection of the organism and insulation. Connective tissue (excluding blood) is found in organs supporting specialised tissues.

The matrix of areolar connective tissue is semi solid, containing adipocytes, mast cells and macrophages. Where there is a need to provide elasticity and tensile strength in the body, areola tissue is present, for example under the skin, between muscles, the alimentary canal. Adipose tissue is found supporting the kidneys, brain and the eyes and is related to energy intake and expenditure. Lymphoid tissue contains reticular cells and white blood cells and is found in lymph tissue in the lymph nodes and all lymphatic organs. Dense connective tissue, fibrous tissue (made up of closely packed collagen fibres with little matrix) is found in ligaments, periosteum, muscle fascia and tendons. Blood is a fluid connective tissue. Cartilage (firmer than other connective tissue) is found as hyaline cartilage on the ends of the bones that form joints, the costal cartilage attaching the ribs to the sternum, forming part of the trachea, larynx and bronchi. Bone cells (the osteocytes) are surrounded by a matrix of collagen fibres with added strength provided by the calcium and phosphate.

Muscle tissue

Muscle tissues are tissues made of cells that permit contractions and as such generate movement. The function of the muscle tissue is to pull bones (skeletal striated muscle), to contract and move viscera and vessels (smooth muscle) as well as making the heart beat (cardiac striated muscle). Each time we move, our heart beats, we breathe, ingest food or urinate, muscle is involved. The muscle cells have internal structures called sarcomeres where there are myosin and actin molecules that work in creating contraction and movement. There are three kinds of muscle in the body: skeletal, cardiac and smooth muscle. Skeletal muscle is also known as striated muscle, it is a voluntary muscle. Cells within the skeletal muscle are long and thin and have multiple nuclei. Cardiac muscle is only found in the heart, it is similar to skeletal muscle with the muscle fibres interlocking with each other ensuring that as one aspect of the muscle is stimulated all other stimulated fibres contact in unison; in a sequential way. Cardiac muscle is not under voluntary control; the special cells of the sino-atrial node are responsible for sending out impulses causing cardiac contraction. Smooth muscle is involuntary and held together by connective tissue with bands of elastic protein wrapped around them. Smooth muscle is found in the walls of hollow structures and vessels, for example, the blood vessels, the ureters, urinary bladder, parts of the respiratory tract, ducts and glands of the alimentary tract.

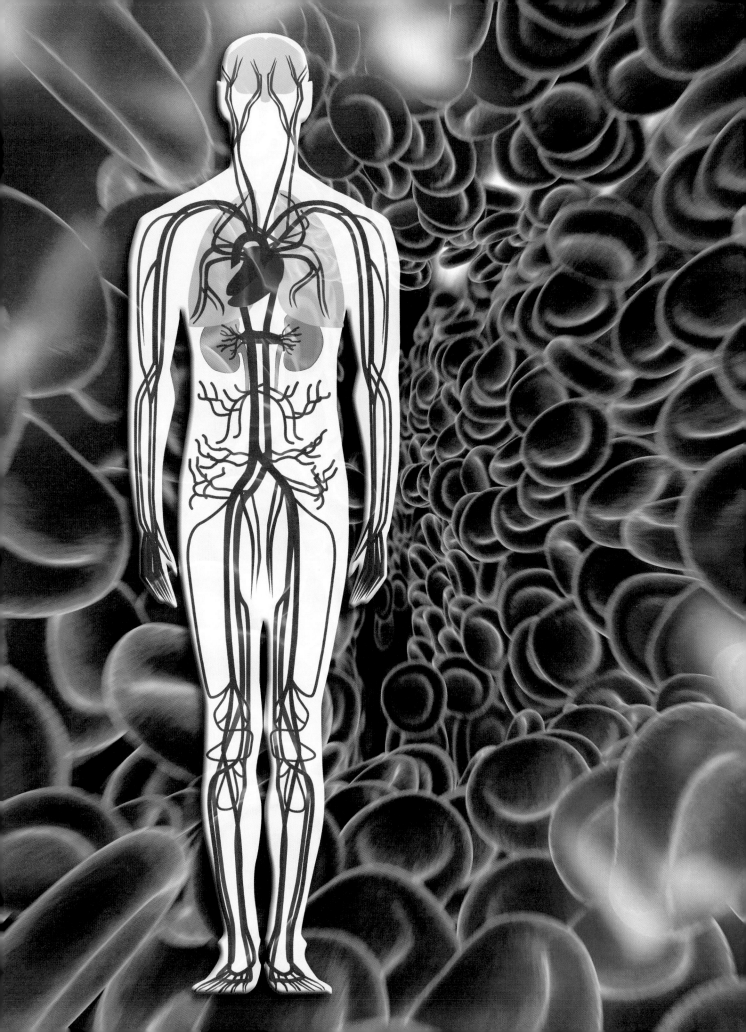

The nervous system

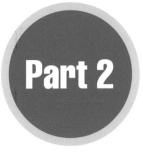

Part 2

Chapters

9 The brain and nerves

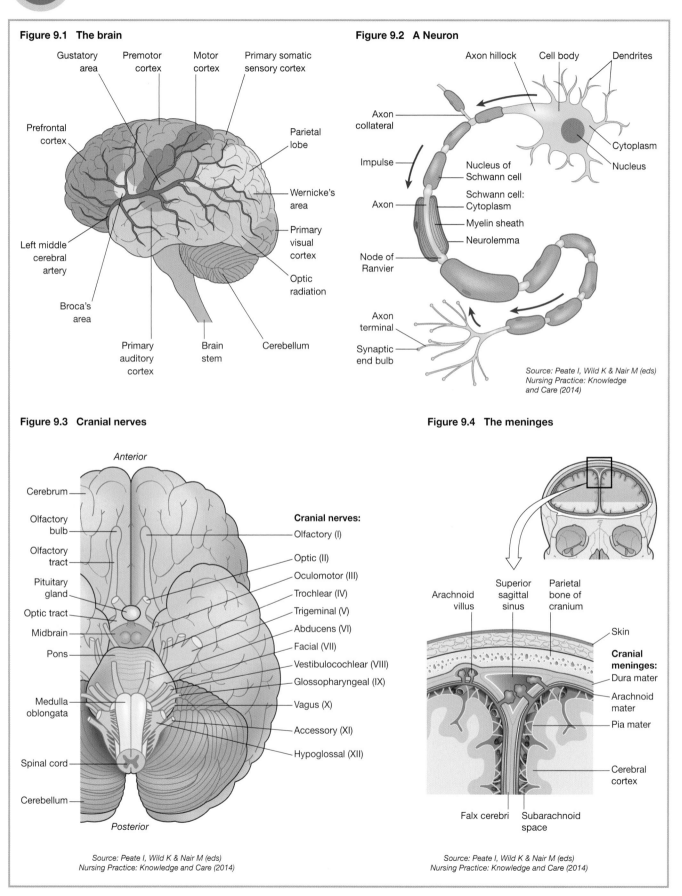

Figure 9.1 The brain

- Gustatory area
- Premotor cortex
- Motor cortex
- Primary somatic sensory cortex
- Prefrontal cortex
- Parietal lobe
- Wernicke's area
- Primary visual cortex
- Left middle cerebral artery
- Optic radiation
- Broca's area
- Primary auditory cortex
- Brain stem
- Cerebellum

Figure 9.2 A Neuron

- Axon hillock
- Cell body
- Dendrites
- Axon collateral
- Cytoplasm
- Impulse
- Nucleus of Schwann cell
- Nucleus
- Axon
- Schwann cell: Cytoplasm
- Myelin sheath
- Neurolemma
- Node of Ranvier
- Axon terminal
- Synaptic end bulb

*Source: Peate I, Wild K & Nair M (eds)
Nursing Practice: Knowledge
and Care (2014)*

Figure 9.3 Cranial nerves

Anterior

- Cerebrum
- Olfactory bulb
- Olfactory tract
- Pituitary gland
- Optic tract
- Midbrain
- Pons
- Medulla oblongata
- Spinal cord
- Cerebellum

Posterior

Cranial nerves:
- Olfactory (I)
- Optic (II)
- Oculomotor (III)
- Trochlear (IV)
- Trigeminal (V)
- Abducens (VI)
- Facial (VII)
- Vestibulocochlear (VIII)
- Glossopharyngeal (IX)
- Vagus (X)
- Accessory (XI)
- Hypoglossal (XII)

*Source: Peate I, Wild K & Nair M (eds)
Nursing Practice: Knowledge and Care (2014)*

Figure 9.4 The meninges

- Arachnoid villus
- Superior sagittal sinus
- Parietal bone of cranium
- Skin
- **Cranial meninges:**
  - Dura mater
  - Arachnoid mater
  - Pia mater
- Cerebral cortex
- Falx cerebri
- Subarachnoid space

*Source: Peate I, Wild K & Nair M (eds)
Nursing Practice: Knowledge and Care (2014)*

Anatomy and Physiology for Nurses at a Glance, First Edition. Ian Peate and Muralitharan Nair. © 2015 John Wiley & Sons, Ltd. Published 2015 by John Wiley & Sons, Ltd.
Companion website: www.ataglanceseries.com/nursing/anatomy

Brain

The human brain (Figure 9.1) has been called the most complex object in the known universe, and in many ways it's the final frontier of science. A hundred billion neurons, and close to a quadrillion connections between them.

The brain lies in the cranial cavity and weighs between 1450–1600 g. It receives 15% of the cardiac output and has a system of autoregulation ensuring the blood supply is constant despite positional changes. Most of the expansion comes from the cerebral cortex, a convoluted layer of neural tissue that covers the surface of the forebrain. Especially expanded are the frontal lobes, which are involved in executive functions such as self-control, planning, reasoning and abstract thought.

Meninges

Nervous tissue is easily damaged by pressure and therefore needs to be protected. The hair, skin and bone offer an outer layer of protection. Adjacent to the nervous tissue are the meninges. The meninges cover the delicate nervous tissue offering protection. They also protect the blood vessels that serve nervous tissue and they contain cerebrospinal fluid. The meninges consist of three connective tissue layers; dura, arachnoid and pia matters (Figure 9.4).

Cerebrospinal fluid

CSF is produced by the choroid plexus in the ventricles of the brain. There is approximately 150 ml of CSF circulating around the brain, in the ventricles and around the spinal cord. The CSF is replaced every 8 hours. The CSF cushions the brain from damage, maintains a uniform pressure between the brain and spinal cord and plays a minor role in fluid and waste exchange between brain and spinal cord.

Neuron

The functional unit of the brain is the neurone or nerve cell (Figure 9.2). It has many features in common with other cells including a nucleus and mitochondria but because of its vital role it is well protected and has some specialist modifications.

Neurones consist of an axon, dendrites and a cell body. Their function is to transmit nerve impulses. Nerve impulses only ever travel in one direction: from the receptive area – the dendrites, to the cell body, and down the length of the axon.

Axon

Each neurone has only one axon, however the axon can branch to form an axon collateral (Figure 9.2). The axon will also branch at its terminal into many axon terminals. The axon length can vary quite significantly from very short to 100 cm long. The axon is considerably thicker and longer than the dendrites of a neuron. Larger neurons have a markedly expanded region at the initial end of the axon called the axon hillock. This axon hillock is the site of summation for incoming information. At any given moment, the collective influence of all neurons that conduct impulses to a given neuron will determine whether or not an action potential will be initiated at the axon hillock and propagated along the axon.

Dendrite

Dendrites are generally very thin appendages that get narrower as they extend further away from the soma (Figure 9.2). Dendritic spines are short outgrowths that further increase the receptive surface area of a neuron. The surface of dendrite branches is covered with junctions that are configured for the reception of incoming information. Dendrites are the short branching processes that receive information. Their branching processes provide a large surface area for this function. In sensory neurones the dendrites often form the part of the sensory receptors and in motor neurones they can be part of the synapse between one neurone and the next.

Cell body

The soma (cell body) is the central part of the neuron. It contains the nucleus of the cell, and therefore is where most protein synthesis occurs. The nucleus ranges from 3 to 18 micrometers in diameter. Most of the neurone cell bodies (Figure 9.2) are located inside the central nervous system and form the grey matter. When clusters of cell bodies are grouped together in the central nervous system they are called nuclei. Cell bodies located in the peripheral nervous system are called ganglia.

Myelin sheath

Oligodendrocytes and Schwann cells form the myelin sheaths that insulate axons in the central and peripheral nervous systems, respectively. Peripheral nerve axons and long or large axons are covered in a myelin sheath (Figure 9.2). Myelin is a fatty material and its purpose is to protect the neurone and to electrically insulate it, speeding up impulse transmission. Within the peripheral nervous system it is Schwann cells wrapped in layers around the neurone that form the myelin sheath. The outermost part of the Schwann cell is its plasma membrane and this is called the neurilemma. There is a regular gap (about 1 mm) between adjacent Schwann cells called the Nodes of Ranvier. Collateral axons can occur at the node. Some nerve fibres are unmyelinated and nerve impulse transmission is significantly slower.

Cranial nerves

The human body contains 12 pairs of cranial nerves that emerge from the brain and supply various structures, most of which are associated with the head and neck (Figure 9.3). The 12 pairs of cranial nerves differ in their functions: some are sensory nerves, that is contain sensory fibres, some are motor nerves, that is contain only motor fibres, and some are mixed nerves, that is contain both sensory and motor nerves.

10 Structures of the brain

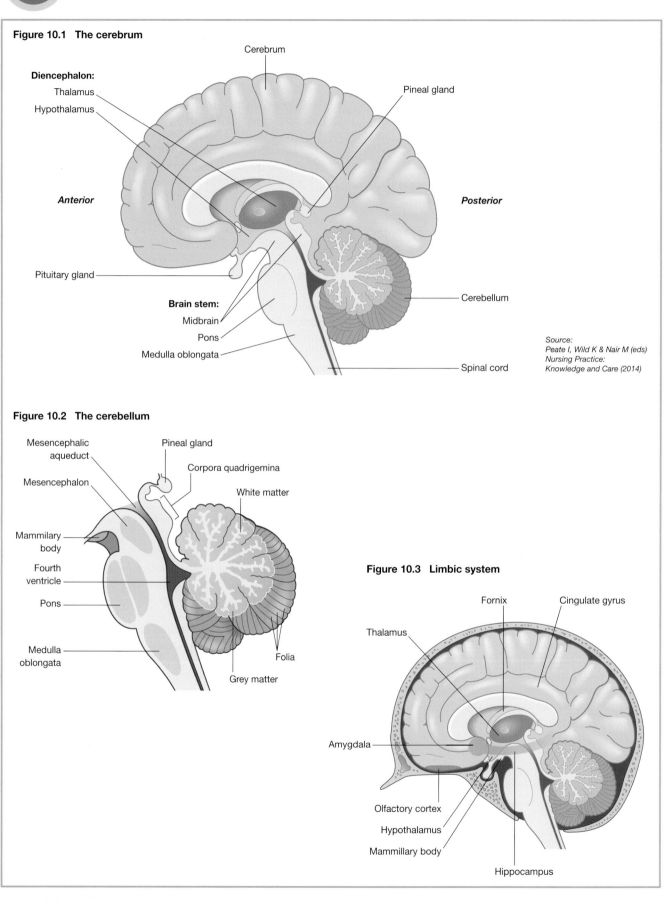

Figure 10.1 The cerebrum

Cerebrum

Diencephalon:
Thalamus
Hypothalamus

Pineal gland

Anterior

Posterior

Pituitary gland

Brain stem:
Midbrain
Pons
Medulla oblongata

Cerebellum

Spinal cord

Source:
Peate I, Wild K & Nair M (eds)
Nursing Practice:
Knowledge and Care (2014)

Figure 10.2 The cerebellum

Mesencephalic aqueduct
Mesencephalon
Mammilary body
Fourth ventricle
Pons
Medulla oblongata

Pineal gland
Corpora quadrigemina
White matter
Folia
Grey matter

Figure 10.3 Limbic system

Fornix
Cingulate gyrus
Thalamus
Amygdala
Olfactory cortex
Hypothalamus
Mammillary body
Hippocampus

Structures of the brain

The brain can be divided into four anatomical regions, each containing one or more structures (Figure 10.1). They include the cerebrum, diencephalon, brain stem and cerebellum.

Cerebrum

The cerebrum, also known as the telencephalon, is the largest and most highly developed part of the human brain. It encompasses about two-thirds of the brain mass and lies over and around most of the structures of the brain (Figure 10.1). The cerebrum of an adult is divided into a pair of large hemispheres. The surfaces of the cerebral hemispheres are highly folded and covered by a superficial layer of grey matter called the cerebral cortex. The functions of the cerebrum include regulation of muscle contraction, memory storage and processing, production of speech, interpretation of taste, sound and memory for storage and processing.

Diencephalon

The diencephalon provides a functional link between the cerebral hemispheres and the rest of the CNS. It contains three paired structures; the thalamus, hypothalamus and the epithalamus.

Thalamus

The thalamus acts as a relay station for sensory impulses going to cerebral cortex for integration and motor impulses entering and leaving the cerebral hemispheres. It also has a role in memory.

Hypothalamus

The hypothalamus is closely associated with the pituitary gland and produces two hormones: antidiuretic hormone (ADH) and oxytocin. It is also the chief autonomic integration centre and is part of the limbic system, which is the emotional brain.

Epithalamus

The epithalamus structure is linked to the pineal gland which secretes the hormone melatonin responsible for sleep wake cycles.

Brain stem

The structures that form the brain stem are involved in many activities that are essential for life. The brain stem is associated with the cranial nerves. The structures of the brain stem include the midbrain, pons and the medulla oblongata (Figure 10.1).

Midbrain

The midbrain contains nuclei that process auditory and visual information and reflexes. It is also maintains consciousness. It provides a conduction pathway that connects the cerebrum with the lower brain structures and spinal cord.

Pons

The pons connects and communicates with the cerebellum. The pons works with the medulla oblongata to control the depth and rate of respiration and contains nuclei that function in visceral and somatic motor control.

Medulla oblongata

The medulla oblongata is a relay station for sensory nerves going to the cerebrum. The medulla contains autonomic centres such as the cardiac centre, the respiratory centre, the vasomotor centre and the coughing, sneezing and vomiting centre. The medulla is also the site of decussation of the pyramidal tracts – this means that the right side of the body is controlled by the left cerebral hemisphere and vice versa.

Cerebellum

Partially hidden by the cerebral hemispheres is the second largest structure of the brain (Figure 10.2). The cerebellum coordinates voluntary muscle movement, motor learning, cognitive functions and balance and posture. It ensures that muscle movements are smooth, coordinated and precise. Motor commands are not initiated in the cerebellum; rather, the cerebellum modifies the motor commands of the descending pathways to make movements more adaptive and accurate. Although the cerebellum accounts for approximately 10% of the brain's volume, it contains over 50% of the total number of neurons in the brain.

Limbic system

The limbic system is a complex set of brain structures that lies on both sides of the thalamus, right under the cerebrum. The limbic system includes the hippocampus, amygdala, anterior thalamic nuclei, septum, habenula, limbic cortex and fornix. It supports a variety of functions, including emotion, behaviour, motivation, long-term memory, and olfaction. The limbic system acts on the endocrine and the autonomic nervous systems.

Ventricles of the brain

The ventricles of the brain are a communicating network of cavities filled with cerebrospinal fluid (CSF) and located within the brain parenchyma. The ventricular system is composed of two lateral ventricles, the third ventricle, the cerebral aqueduct, and the fourth ventricle (see the following images). The choroid plexuses located in the ventricles produce CSF, which fills the ventricles and subarachnoid space, following a cycle of constant production and reabsorption.

Cerebrospinal fluid

The ventricles are filled with cerebrospinal fluid (CSF) which bathes and cushions the brain and spinal cord within their bony confines. Cerebrospinal fluid is produced by modified ependymal cells of the choroid plexus found in all components of the ventricular system except for the cerebral aqueduct and the posterior and anterior horns of the lateral ventricles. CSF flows from the lateral ventricle to the third ventricle through the interventricular foramen (also called the foramen of Monro). The third ventricle and fourth ventricle are connected to each other by the cerebral aqueduct (also called the Aqueduct of Sylvius). CSF then flows into the subarachnoid space through the foramina of Luschka (there are two of these) and the foramen of Magendie (only one of these).

There is approximately 150 ml of CSF circulating around the brain, in the ventricles and around the spinal cord. The CSF is replaced every 8 hours. Absorption of the CSF into the blood stream takes place in the superior sagittal sinus through structures called arachnoid villi. When the CSF pressure is greater than the venous pressure, CSF will flow into the blood stream. However, the arachnoid villi act as 'one way valves': if the CSF pressure is less than the venous pressure, the arachnoid villi will **NOT** let blood pass into the ventricular system.

11 The spinal cord

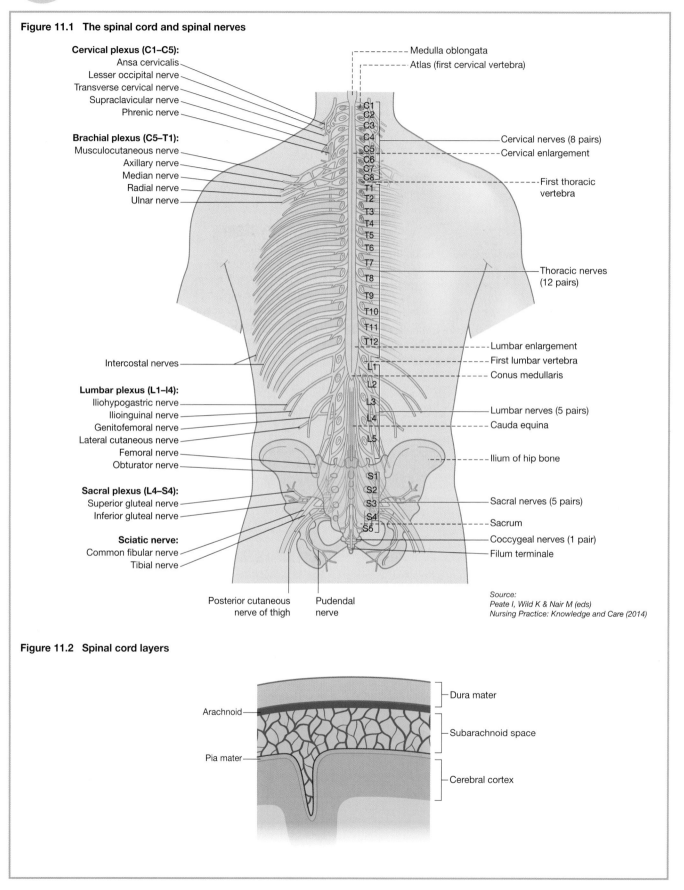

Figure 11.1 The spinal cord and spinal nerves

Cervical plexus (C1–C5):
Ansa cervicalis
Lesser occipital nerve
Transverse cervical nerve
Supraclavicular nerve
Phrenic nerve

Brachial plexus (C5–T1):
Musculocutaneous nerve
Axillary nerve
Median nerve
Radial nerve
Ulnar nerve

Intercostal nerves

Lumbar plexus (L1–I4):
Iliohypogastric nerve
Ilioinguinal nerve
Genitofemoral nerve
Lateral cutaneous nerve
Femoral nerve
Obturator nerve

Sacral plexus (L4–S4):
Superior gluteal nerve
Inferior gluteal nerve

Sciatic nerve:
Common fibular nerve
Tibial nerve

Posterior cutaneous nerve of thigh

Pudendal nerve

Medulla oblongata
Atlas (first cervical vertebra)

Cervical nerves (8 pairs)
Cervical enlargement

First thoracic vertebra

Thoracic nerves (12 pairs)

Lumbar enlargement
First lumbar vertebra
Conus medullaris

Lumbar nerves (5 pairs)
Cauda equina

Ilium of hip bone

Sacral nerves (5 pairs)

Sacrum
Coccygeal nerves (1 pair)
Filum terminale

Source:
Peate I, Wild K & Nair M (eds)
Nursing Practice: Knowledge and Care (2014)

Figure 11.2 Spinal cord layers

Arachnoid
Pia mater

Dura mater
Subarachnoid space
Cerebral cortex

Anatomy and Physiology for Nurses at a Glance, First Edition. Ian Peate and Muralitharan Nair. © 2015 John Wiley & Sons, Ltd. Published 2015 by John Wiley & Sons, Ltd.
Companion website: www.ataglanceseries.com/nursing/anatomy

Spinal cord

The adult spinal cord is approximately 45 cm in length and 14 mm in width (Figure 11.1). There are two layers; an outer layer of white matter and in inner layer made up of grey matter, which surrounds a small central canal. The spinal cord is enclosed within the vertebral canal which forms a protective ring of bone around the cord. Other protective coverings include the spinal meninges, which are three layers of connective tissue coverings which extend around the spinal cord. The spinal meninges consist of pia matter (inner layer), arachnoid matter (middle layer) and dura matter (the outermost layer which consists of a dense, irregular connective tissue).

Pia matter

Pia matter, often referred to as simply the pia, is the delicate innermost layer of the meninges, the membranes surrounding the brain and spinal cord (Figure 11.2). Pia matter is the thin, translucent, mesh-like meningeal envelope, spanning nearly the entire surface of the brain. The pia is firmly adhered to the surface of the brain and loosely connected to the arachnoid layer. The pia matter functions to cover and protect the CNS, to protect the blood vessels and enclose the venous sinuses near the CNS, to contain the cerebrospinal fluid (CSF) and to form partitions with the skull.

Arachnoid matter

The arachnoid matter is the protective membrane that covers the brain and spinal cord (Figure 11.2). It includes a simple squamous epithelium called the arachnoid membrane and the arachnoid trabeculae which is a network of collagen elastic fibres that extend between the arachnoid membrane and the outer surface of the pia matter.

Dura matter

The dura matter is a thin membrane that is the outermost of the three layers of the meninges that surround the brain and spinal cord (Figure 11.2). The dura matter has several functions and layers. The dura matter is a sac that envelops the arachnoid matter. It surrounds and supports the dural sinuses and carries blood from the brain toward the heart.

Spinal cord sections

The human spinal cord is divided into 31 different segments. At every segment, right and left pairs of spinal nerves (mixed: sensory and motor) form. Six to eight motor nerve rootlets branch out of right and left ventro lateral sulci in a very orderly manner. Nerve rootlets combine to form nerve roots.

Each segment of the spinal cord is associated with a pair of ganglia, called dorsal root ganglia, which are situated just outside of the spinal cord. These ganglia contain cell bodies of sensory neurons. Axons of these sensory neurons travel into the spinal cord via the dorsal roots.

The spinal cord is supplied with blood by three arteries that run along its length starting in the brain, and many arteries that approach it through the sides of the spinal column. The three longitudinal arteries are called the anterior spinal artery, and the right and left posterior spinal arteries. These travel in the subarachnoid space and send branches into the spinal cord.

Functions of the spinal cord

The spinal cord provides a means of communication between the brain and the peripheral nerves that leave the spinal cord and has two major functions in maintaining homeostasis:
- The tracts of the white matter of the spinal cord carry sensory impulses to the brain and motor impulses from the brain to the skeletal muscles and other effector muscles.
- The grey matter, in the centre of the cord, is shaped like a butterfly and consists of cell bodies of interneurons and motor neurons. The grey matter is a site for integration of reflexes, which is a rapid, involuntary action in relation to a particular stimulus.

Reflex actions

Spinal cord controls some other important functions, such as reflex actions. For reflex actions, the spinal cord does not take any assistance from the brain. Reflex actions are automatic, unlearned, involuntary and inborn responses. Therefore, these actions are sudden in nature and have a purpose of protecting the individual from sudden danger.

For example, if someone throws a stone towards you; suddenly you move your body to avoid the incoming danger of being hurt. The path through which reflex action is conducted is known as the 'reflex arc', which involves (i) receptor, (ii) afferent neuron, (iii) spinal cord, (iv) inter-neuron, (v) efferent neuron, (vi) muscles or gland.

Spinal nerves

There are 31 pairs of spinal nerves attached to the spinal cord within the human body which are named and numbered according to the region and level of the vertebral column from which they emerge. Each nerve innervates a group of muscles (myotome) and an area of skin (dermatome) and most also innervate some of the thoracic and abdominal organs.

The spinal nerves provide the paths of communication between the spinal cord and specific regions of the body as they connect the CNS to sensory receptors, muscles and glands in all the parts of the body. A typical spinal nerve has two connections to the spinal cord: a posterior root and an anterior root which unite to form a spinal nerve at the intervertebral foramen. A spinal nerve is an example of a mixed nerve as it contains both sensory (posterior root) and motor (anterior root) nerves.

12 The blood supply

Figure 12.1 Circle of Willis

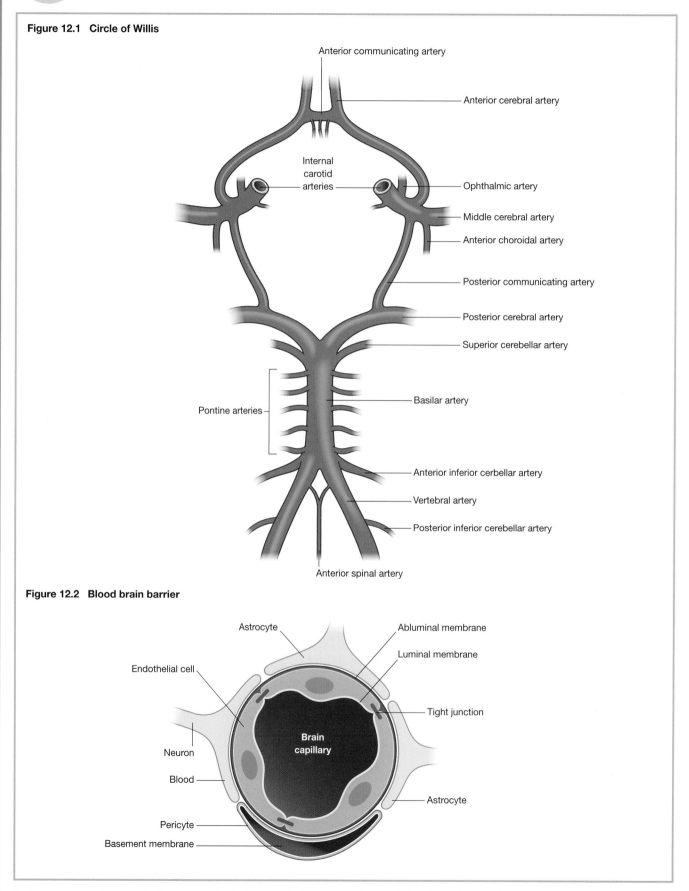

Anterior communicating artery

Anterior cerebral artery

Internal carotid arteries

Ophthalmic artery

Middle cerebral artery

Anterior choroidal artery

Posterior communicating artery

Posterior cerebral artery

Superior cerebellar artery

Pontine arteries

Basilar artery

Anterior inferior cerbellar artery

Vertebral artery

Posterior inferior cerebellar artery

Anterior spinal artery

Figure 12.2 Blood brain barrier

Astrocyte

Abluminal membrane

Luminal membrane

Endothelial cell

Tight junction

Brain capillary

Neuron

Blood

Astrocyte

Pericyte

Basement membrane

Anatomy and Physiology for Nurses at a Glance, First Edition. Ian Peate and Muralitharan Nair. © 2015 John Wiley & Sons, Ltd. Published 2015 by John Wiley & Sons, Ltd.
Companion website: www.ataglanceseries.com/nursing/anatomy

Circle of Willis

The circle of Willis (circulus arteriosus cerebri) is an anastomotic system of arteries (Figure 12.1) that sits at the base of the brain. The 'circle' was named after Thomas Willis by his student Richard Lower. Willis was the author of *Cerebri Anatome,* a book that described and depicted this vascular ring. Although such a vascular ring had been described earlier, the name Willis has been eponymously propagated.

The circle of Willis encircles the stalk of the pituitary gland and provides important communications between the blood supply of the forebrain and hindbrain. The circle of Willis is formed when the internal carotid artery enters the cranial cavity bilaterally and divides into the anterior cerebral artery and middle cerebral artery.

The anterior cerebral arteries are then united by an anterior communicating artery. These connections form the anterior half (anterior circulation) of the circle of Willis. Posteriorly, the basilar artery, formed by the left and right vertebral arteries, branches into a left and right posterior cerebral artery, forming the posterior circulation. The PCAs complete the circle of Willis by joining the internal carotid system anteriorly via the posterior communicating arteries.

Although in an adult the brain represents only 2% of the total body weight, it utilises 20% of oxygen and glucose even at rest. When activities in a certain area of the brain increase, blood flow to that region also increases. Even a brief slowing of blood flow to the brain can result in unconsciousness.

Further decrease in blood flow, for a couple of minutes, can lead to impaired neuronal function. If the blood flow is restricted for four minutes or more then it could lead to permanent brain damage. As the brain does not store glucose there must be a continuous supply of glucose to the brain.

Function of the circle of Willis

The circle of Willis provides multiple paths for oxygenated blood to supply the brain if any of the principal suppliers of oxygenated blood (i.e. the vertebral and internal carotid arteries) are constricted by physical pressure, occluded by disease, or interrupted by injury. This redundancy of blood supply is generally termed collateral circulation.

Blood–brain barrier (BBB)

The BBB is semi-permeable; that is, it allows some materials to cross, but prevents others from crossing. In most parts of the body, the smallest blood vessels, called capillaries, are lined with endothelial cells. Endothelial tissue has small spaces between each individual cell so substances can move readily between the inside and the outside of the vessel. However, in the brain, the endothelial cells fit tightly together and substances cannot pass out of the bloodstream (Figure 12.2). (Some molecules, such as glucose, are transported out of the blood by special methods.)

Glial cells (astrocytes) form a layer around brain blood vessels and may be important in the development of the BBB. Astrocytes may be also be responsible for transporting ions from the brain to the blood.

Function of BBB

The existence of BBB protects brain cells from harmful substances and pathogens by preventing passage of many substances from the blood into the brain tissue. It also provides a constant environment for the brain and protects the brain from hormones and neurotransmitters in the rest of the body.

A few water soluble substances, such as glucose, cross the BBB by active transport. Other substances such as urea and most ions cross the BBB very slowly. Protein and most antibiotics do not cross the BBB to get into the brain tissue. However, lipid soluble substances such as oxygen, carbon dioxide, alcohol and most anaesthetic drugs cross the BBB easily.

The BBB can be broken down by hypertension (high blood pressure): high blood pressure opens the BBB. Exposure to microwaves, exposure to radiation, infection and injury to the brain such as trauma, inflammation and ischaemia can all open the BBB. The BBB is not considered to affect the movement of inflammatory cells into the CNS; activated lymphocytes can enter the normal CNS.

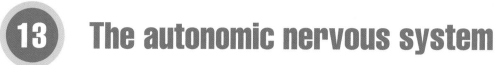

13 The autonomic nervous system

Figure 13.1 The sympathetic and parasympathetic nervous system

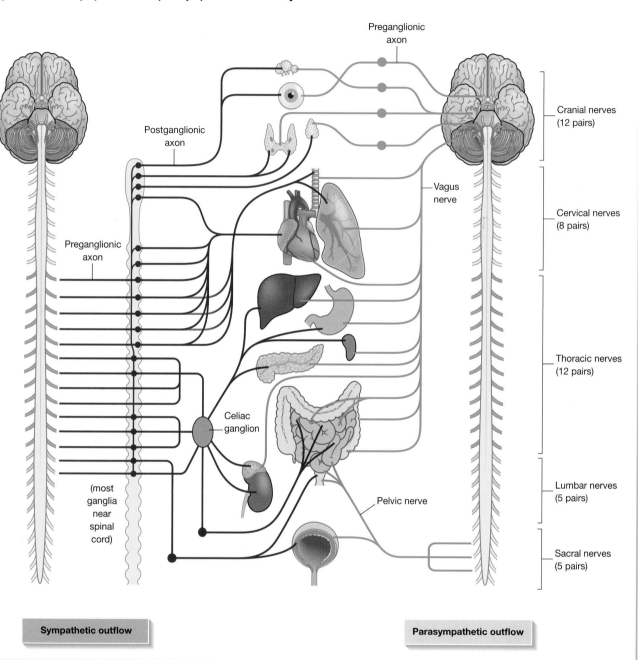

Anatomy and Physiology for Nurses at a Glance, First Edition. Ian Peate and Muralitharan Nair. © 2015 John Wiley & Sons, Ltd. Published 2015 by John Wiley & Sons, Ltd.
Companion website: www.ataglanceseries.com/nursing/anatomy

ANS

The autonomic nervous system (ANS) plays a major role in the maintenance of homeostasis by regulating the body's automatic, involuntary functions, and in common with the rest of the nervous system consists of neurones, neuroglia and other connective tissue. However its structure is quite unique in that it is divided into two, namely the sympathetic division and the parasympathetic division. Most autonomic responses cannot be consciously altered or suppressed to any great degree.

Sympathetic nervous system

The sympathetic division includes nerve fibres that arise from the 12 thoracic and first two lumbar segments of the spinal cord, hence it is also referred to as the thoracicolumbar division. The sympathetic division takes control of many internal organs when a stressful situation occurs. This can take the form of physical stress for example if undertaking strenuous exercise, or emotional stress such as at times of anger or anxiety. In emergency situations, the sympathetic nervous system releases norepinephrine which assists in the 'fight or flight' response.

Like other parts of the nervous system, the sympathetic nervous system operates through a series of interconnected neurons. Sympathetic neurons are frequently considered part of the peripheral nervous system (PNS), although there are many that lie within the central nervous system (CNS). Sympathetic neurons of the spinal cord (which is part of the CNS) communicate with peripheral sympathetic neurons via a series of sympathetic ganglia. Within the ganglia, spinal cord sympathetic neurons join peripheral sympathetic neurons through chemical synapses.

Spinal cord sympathetic neurons are therefore called presynaptic (or preganglionic) neurons, while peripheral sympathetic neurons are called postsynaptic (or postganglionic) neurons. At synapses within the sympathetic ganglia, preganglionic sympathetic neurons release acetylcholine, a chemical messenger that binds and activates nicotinic acetylcholine receptors on postganglionic neurons.

Functions

Nerves of the sympathetic division speed up heart rate, dilate pupils, relax the bladder, increase blood pressure, increase respiration, dilate blood vessels to heart, increase blood flow to muscles, release epinephrine, release stored energy (glycogen), increase perspiration, decrease blood to skin and slow down the GI tract.

Parasympathetic nervous system

The parasympathetic division includes fibres that arise from the lower end of the spinal cord and includes several cranial nerves – hence it is often referred to as the craniosacral division. The parasympathetic division is most active when the body is at rest and utilises acetylcholine to control all the internal responses associated with a state of relaxation (Figure 13.1) and therefore has many opposite effects on the body to the sympathetic nervous system.

In contract to the 'flight or fight' activities of the sympathetic division, the parasympathetic division enhances 'rest and digest'. The parasympathetic responses support body functions that conserve and restore body energy during times of rest and recovery.

The parasympathetic nervous system is composed of four cranial nerves that originate from the brainstem. The PNS activity begins in the head in the sacral region, this is why this activity is called cranio-sacral in nature while the SNS is thoraco-lumbar in nature. The most involved nerve in a PNS activity is the vagus nerve. It works by transmitting information between the posterior hypothalamus, the brainstem of the central nervous system and vital organs as well as the glands. The sympathetic nervous system does the fight and flight functions, while the parasympathetic nervous system performs the rest and digest responses. PNS works by antagonising the action of SNS by lowering heart rate, decreasing blood pressure, constricting pupils and increasing intestinal motility. It increases the release of endorphins, a hormone that is called 'feel good,' so we can recover from the actions from sympathetic nervous system stimulation.

Functions

- decreases HR and BP
- slows breathing
- lubricates mouth, eyes
- stimulates digestion and storing energy
- constricts pupil
- responsible for elimination

Autonomic control by the CNS

The hypothalamus is the major control and integration centre of the ANS. The hypothalamus receives sensory input related to visceral function, smell, taste, temperature and osmolality of blood. It also receives information about the emotional feeling from the limbic system. The output from the hypothalamus influences the autonomic centres both in the brain stem (cardiac, respiration, salivation centres) and the spinal cord (defecation, urination reflex centres).

Anatomically, the hypothalamus is connected both to the sympathetic and the parasympathetic divisions. For example, stimulation of the sympathetic division increases the heart rate and the parasympathetic division reduces the heart rate.

Autonomic reflexes

Autonomic reflexes are responses that occur when nerve impulses pass through an autonomic reflex arc. These play an important part in regulating controlled conditions in the body, for example blood pressure regulation takes place by altering heart rate, force of ventricular contraction and vascular diameter.

The components for an autonomic reflex arc include a receptor (responds to a stimulus and produces a change that will ultimately trigger nerve impulses), sensory neuron (conduct nerve impulses from receptors to the CNS), integrating centre (located in the hypothalamus and spinal cord), motor neurons (impulses from CNS along the motor neurone to the effector) and an effector (smooth muscle, cardiac muscle and glands).

14 Peripheral nervous system

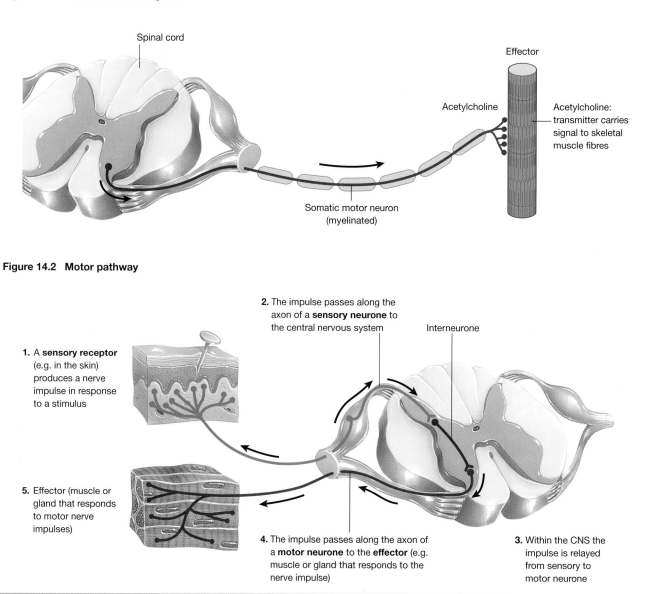

Figure 14.1 Somatic nervous system

Spinal cord

Effector

Acetylcholine

Acetylcholine: transmitter carries signal to skeletal muscle fibres

Somatic motor neuron (myelinated)

Figure 14.2 Motor pathway

1. A **sensory receptor** (e.g. in the skin) produces a nerve impulse in response to a stimulus

2. The impulse passes along the axon of a **sensory neurone** to the central nervous system

Interneurone

5. Effector (muscle or gland that responds to motor nerve impulses)

4. The impulse passes along the axon of a **motor neurone** to the **effector** (e.g. muscle or gland that responds to the nerve impulse)

3. Within the CNS the impulse is relayed from sensory to motor neurone

PNS

The peripheral nervous system includes all the tissues that lie outside the CNS. These include cranial nerves, spinal cord, spinal nerves and autonomic system (see Chapter 13). There are two types of cells in the peripheral nervous system. These cells carry information to (sensory nervous cells) and from (motor nervous cells) the central nervous system (CNS). Cells of the sensory nervous system send information to the CNS from internal organs or from external stimuli.

Motor nervous system cells carry information from the CNS to organs, muscles and glands. The motor nervous system is divided into the somatic nervous system and the autonomic nervous system. The somatic nervous system controls skeletal muscle as well as external sensory organs such as the skin. This system is said to be voluntary because the responses can be controlled consciously. Reflex reactions of skeletal muscle however are an exception. These are involuntary reactions to external stimuli.

Peripheral nervous system connections

Peripheral nervous system connections with various organs and structures of the body are established through cranial nerves and spinal nerves. There are 12 pairs of cranial nerves (see Chapter 9) in the brain that establish connections in the head and upper body, while 31 pairs of spinal nerves (see Chapter 11) do the same for the rest of the body. While some cranial nerves contain only sensory neurons, most cranial nerves and all spinal nerves contain both motor and sensory neurons.

Sensory division

The sensory (afferent) division carries sensory signals by way of afferent nerve fibres from receptors in the central nervous system (CNS). It can be further subdivided into somatic and visceral divisions. The somatic sensory division carries signals from receptors in the skin, muscles, bones and joints. The visceral sensory division carries signals mainly from the viscera of the thoracic and abdominal cavities.

Somatic

The somatic nervous system (SNS) (Figure 14.1) is the portion of the nervous system responsible for voluntary body movement and for sensing external stimuli. All five senses are controlled by this system. The SNS is a sub-part of the peripheral nervous system.

The SNS enervates all sensory organs, including the eyes, ears, tongue and skin, as well as all the skeletal muscles, and the muscles attached to the bone and used for voluntary movement. In movement, the SNS carries impulses from the brain to the muscle to be moved, while in its sensory capacity, the SNS carries impulses from the sensory organ to the brain. There are therefore two portions, or limbs, of the somatic nervous system, the afferent and the efferent. The afferent, or sensory, neurons carry impulses from sense organs into the central nervous system, while the efferent, or motor, neurons carry impulses from the central nervous system to the muscles.

Visceral

The visceral division supplies and receives fibres to and from smooth muscle, cardiac muscle and glands. The visceral motor fibres (those supplying smooth muscle, cardiac muscle, and glands) make up the autonomic nervous system (see Chapter 13). The ANS has two divisions:
- Parasympathetic division – important for control of 'normal' body functions, such as normal operation of digestive system.
- Sympathetic division – also called the 'fight or flight' division; important in helping us cope with stress.

Motor division

The motor (efferent) division carries motor signals by way of efferent nerve fibres from the CNS to effectors (mainly glands and muscles) (Figure 14.2). It can be further divided into somatic and visceral divisions. The somatic motor division carries signals to the skeletal muscles. The visceral motor division, also known as the autonomic nervous system, carries signals to glands, cardiac muscle and smooth muscle. It can be further subdivided into the sympathetic and parasympathetic divisions (see Chapter 13).

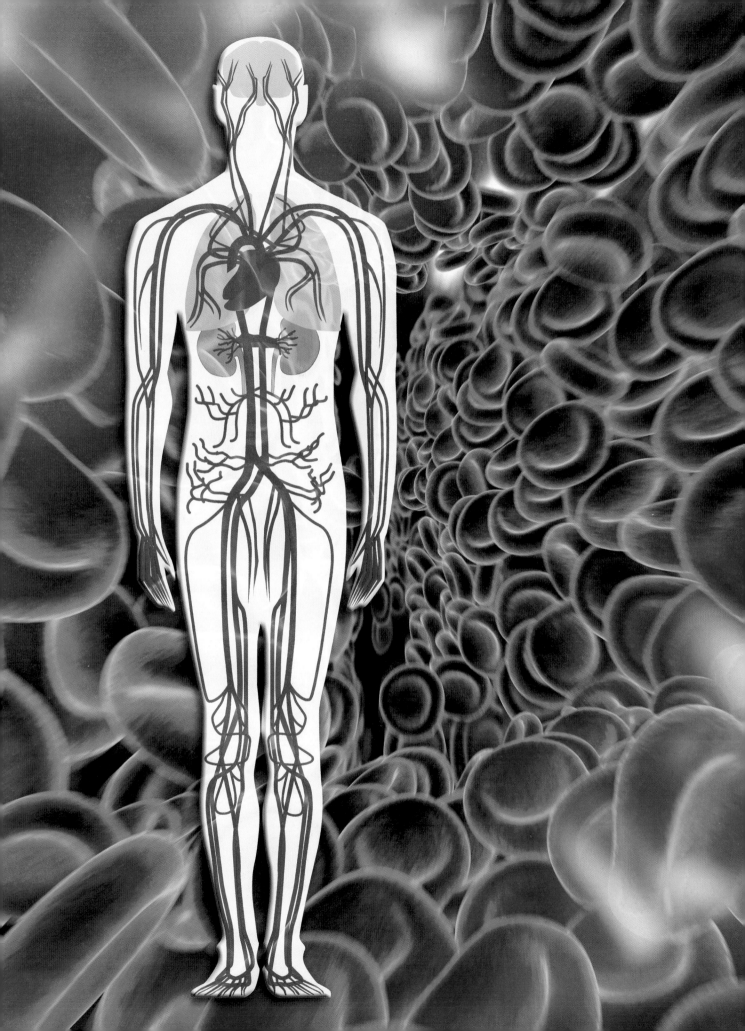

The heart and vascular system

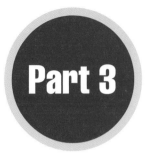

Part 3

Chapters

15 The heart

Figure 15.1 Location of the heart

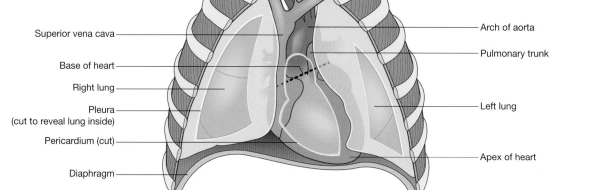

Superior vena cava

Base of heart

Right lung

Pleura
(cut to reveal lung inside)

Pericardium (cut)

Diaphragm

Arch of aorta

Pulmonary trunk

Left lung

Apex of heart

Source: Peate I, Wild K & Nair M (eds) Nursing Practice: Knowledge and Care (2014)

Figure 15.2 Walls of the heart

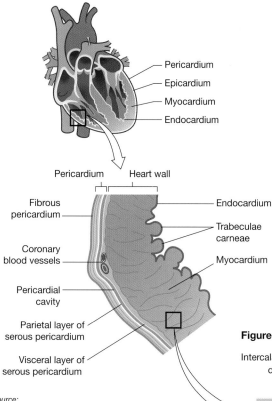

Pericardium
Epicardium
Myocardium
Endocardium

Pericardium | Heart wall

Fibrous
pericardium

Coronary
blood vessels

Pericardial
cavity

Parietal layer of
serous pericardium

Visceral layer of
serous pericardium

Endocardium

Trabeculae
carneae

Myocardium

Source:
Peate I, Wild K & Nair M (eds)
Nursing Practice: Knowledge
and Care (2014)

Figure 15.4 Chambers of the heart

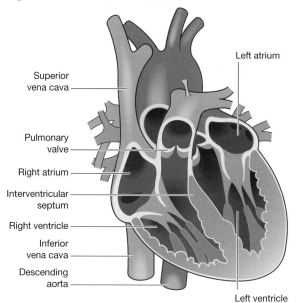

Left atrium

Superior
vena cava

Pulmonary
valve

Right atrium

Interventricular
septum

Right ventricle

Inferior
vena cava

Descending
aorta

Left ventricle

Source: Peate I, Wild K & Nair M (eds) Nursing Practice: Knowledge and Care (2014)

Figure 15.3 Myocardium cells

Intercalated
discs

Cross-
striations

Nuclei

Myocytes

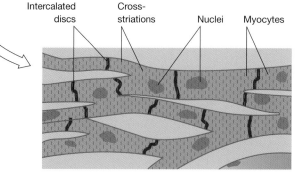

Source:
Peate I & Nair M Fundamentals
of Anatomy and Physiology for
Student Nurses (2011)

Heart

The heart weighs about 250–390 g in men and 200–275 g women and is a little larger than the owner's closed fist, being approximately 12 cm long and 9 cm wide. It is located in the thoracic cavity (chest) in the mediastinum (between the lungs), behind and to the left of the sternum (breast bone) (Figure 15.1). The heart rests on the diaphragm in the thoracic cavity.

Walls of the heart

Pericardium

The heart is surrounded by a membrane called the pericardium (peri = around), this is often referred to as a single sac surrounding the heart but is in fact made up of two sacs (the fibrous pericardium and the serous pericardium) that are closely connected to each other (Figure 15.2). These two sacs have very different structure.

Fibrous pericardium

A tough, inelastic, layer made up of dense, irregular, connective tissue. The role of this layer is to prevent the overstretching of the heart. It also provides protection to the heart and anchors it in place.

Parietal pericardium

The serous pericardium is a thinner, more delicate, layer that forms a double layer around the heart. This outer layer is fused to the fibrous pericardium. The visceral pericardium (otherwise known as the epicardium) adheres tightly to the surface of the heart.

Myocardium

The myocardium makes up the majority of the bulk of the heart. It is a specialised muscle only found within the heart and is specialised in its structure and function. The myocardium can be divided into two categories: the majority specialised to perform mechanical work (contraction); the remainder specialised to the task of initiating and conducting electrical impulses. The cardiac muscle cells (myocytes) are held together in interlacing bundles of fibres that are arranged in a spiral or circular bundles (Figure 15.3).

Myocardial thickness varies between the four chambers. The ventricles have thicker walls then the atria; however, the left ventricle has the thickest myocardial wall. This is because the left ventricle pumps blood great distances to parts of the body at a higher pressure and the resistance to blood flow is greater.

Endocardium

The innermost layer made up of endothelium overlaying a thin layer of connective tissue. The endothelium is continuous with the endothelial lining of the large vessels of the heart. It also provides a smooth lining for the blood to flow through the chambers smoothly.

Chambers of the heart

The heart has four chambers, two atria (left and right) and two ventricles (left and right). On the anterior surface of each atrium is a wrinkled pouch-like structure called an auricle. The main function of the auricle is to increase the volume of blood in the atrium. Between the ventricles is a dividing wall, the intraventricular septum (Figure 15.4). Thus with the septum between the atria and the septum between the ventricles there is no mixing of blood between the two sides.

Valves of the heart

Between the atria and the ventricles are two valves (the atrioventricular valves).
- The tricuspid valve – this is made up of three cusps (leaflets) and lies between the right atrium and the right ventricle.
- The bicuspid (mitral) valve – this is made up of two cusps and lies between the left atrium and the left ventricle.

The purpose of the atrioventricular valves is to prevent the backward flow of blood from the ventricles into the atria.

Blood vessels of the heart

The aorta is the largest blood vessel of the heart. The aorta carries and distributes oxygen-rich blood to all arteries. The coronary arteries are the first blood vessels that branch off from the ascending aorta. The coronary arteries supply oxygenated and nutrient filled blood to the heart muscle. There are two main coronary arteries: the right coronary artery and left coronary artery. Other arteries diverge from these two main arteries and extend to the bottom portion of the heart.

The pulmonary arteries are unique in that unlike most arteries which carry oxygenated blood to other parts of the body, the pulmonary arteries carry de-oxygenated blood to the lungs. After picking up oxygen, the oxygen-rich blood is returned to the heart via the pulmonary veins.

There are four pulmonary veins which extend from the left atrium to the lungs. They are the right superior, right inferior, left superior and left inferior pulmonary veins.

The venae cavae (superior and inferior) are the two largest veins in the body. These blood vessels carry de-oxygenated blood from various regions of the body to the right atrium of the heart. As the de-oxygenated blood is returned to the heart and continues to flow through the cardiac cycle, it is transported to the lungs where it becomes oxygenated. The blood then travels back to the heart and is pumped out to the rest of the body via the aorta. Oxygen depleted blood is returned to the heart again via the venae cavae.

16 Blood flow through the heart

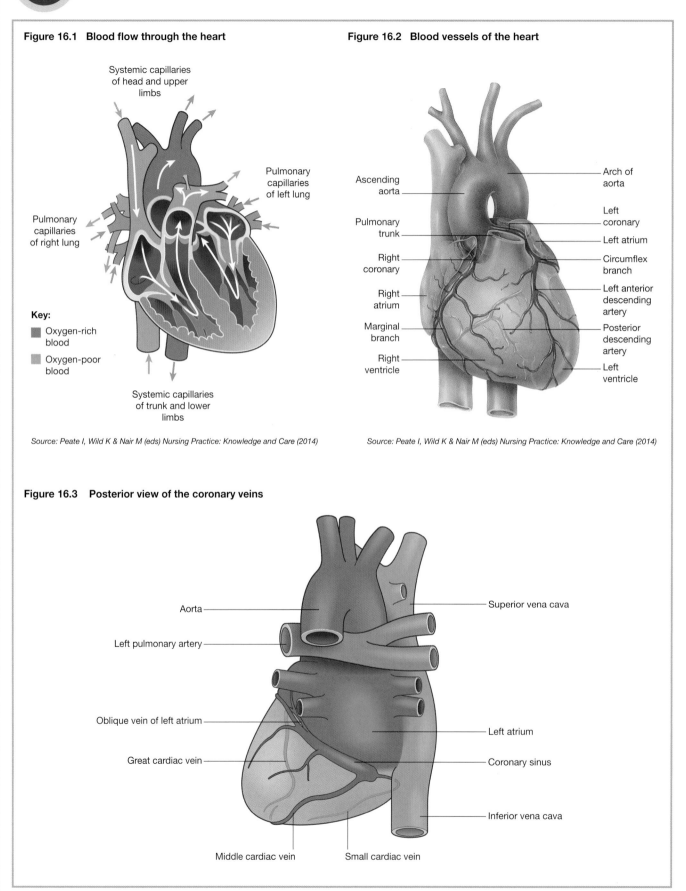

Figure 16.1 Blood flow through the heart

Systemic capillaries
of head and upper
limbs

Pulmonary
capillaries
of left lung

Pulmonary
capillaries
of right lung

Key:

■ Oxygen-rich
blood

■ Oxygen-poor
blood

Systemic capillaries
of trunk and lower
limbs

Source: Peate I, Wild K & Nair M (eds) Nursing Practice: Knowledge and Care (2014)

Figure 16.2 Blood vessels of the heart

Ascending
aorta

Pulmonary
trunk

Right
coronary

Right
atrium

Marginal
branch

Right
ventricle

Arch of
aorta

Left
coronary

Left atrium

Circumflex
branch

Left anterior
descending
artery

Posterior
descending
artery

Left
ventricle

Source: Peate I, Wild K & Nair M (eds) Nursing Practice: Knowledge and Care (2014)

Figure 16.3   Posterior view of the coronary veins

Aorta

Left pulmonary artery

Oblique vein of left atrium

Great cardiac vein

Middle cardiac vein

Small cardiac vein

Superior vena cava

Left atrium

Coronary sinus

Inferior vena cava

Blood flow

The body's circulatory system really has three distinct parts: pulmonary circulation, coronary circulation and systemic circulation, in other words, the lungs (pulmonary), the heart (coronary) and the rest of the system (systemic) circulation. Each part must be working independently in order for them to all work together.

Pulmonary circulation

Pulmonary circulation is a system of blood vessels that forms a closed circuit between the heart and the lungs.

Blood enters the heart through two large veins, the inferior and superior vena cava, emptying oxygen-poor blood from the body into the right atrium. Blood flows from the right atrium into your right ventricle through the open tricuspid valve. When the ventricles are full, the tricuspid valve shuts. This prevents blood from flowing backward into the atria while the ventricles contract (squeeze).

Once blood travels through the pulmonary valve, it enters the lungs. This is called the pulmonary circulation. From the pulmonary valve, blood travels to the pulmonary artery to tiny capillary vessels in the lungs. Here, oxygen travels from the tiny air sacs in the lungs, through the walls of the capillaries, into the blood. At the same time, carbon dioxide, a waste product of metabolism, passes from the blood into the air sacs. Carbon dioxide leaves the body when we exhale. Once the blood is purified and oxygenated, it travels back to the left atrium through the pulmonary veins (Figure 16.1).

Systemic circulation

The systemic circulation is the circuit of vessels supplying oxygenated blood to and returning deoxygenated blood from the tissues of the body. The pulmonary vein empties oxygen-rich blood, from the lungs into the left atrium.

Blood leaves the heart through the aortic valve, into the aorta and to the body. This pattern is repeated, causing blood to flow continuously to the heart, lungs and body (Figure 16.1).

The forceful contraction of the heart's left ventricle forces the blood into the aorta which then branches into many smaller arteries which run throughout the body. The inside layer of an artery is very smooth, allowing the blood to flow quickly. The outside layer of an artery is very strong, allowing the blood to flow forcefully. The oxygen-rich blood enters the capillaries where the oxygen and nutrients are released. The waste products are collected and the waste-rich blood flows into the veins in order to circulate back to the heart where pulmonary circulation will allow the exchange of gases in the lungs.

Coronary circulation

The heart receives about 5% of the body's blood supply. Ensuring that the heart receives a plentiful supply of blood is essential to ensure the constant supply of oxygen and nutrients and the efficient removal of waste products required by the myocardium.

Nutrients from the blood cannot diffuse quickly from the chambers to supply the cells of the heart. Only the inner part of the endocardium (about 2 mm in thickness) is supplied with blood directly from the inside of the heart chambers. The rest of the heart is supplied by the coronary arteries. The coronary arteries come directly off the aorta, just after the aortic valve. They continuously divide into smaller branches, forming a web of blood vessels to supply the heart muscle (Figure 16.2).

Coronary arteries

Coronary arteries supply blood to the heart muscle. Like all other tissues in the body, the heart muscle needs oxygen-rich blood to function, and oxygen-depleted blood must be carried away.

The coronary arteries branch from the ascending aorta and encircle the heart like a crown. As the coronary arteries are compressed during each heart beat blood does not flow through the coronary arteries at this time. Thus blood flow to the myocardium occurs during the relaxation phase, this is the opposite of every other part of the body.

The left coronary artery divides into the anterior interventricular, branch, which supplies oxygenated blood to both ventricles, and the circumflex branch, which distributes oxygenated blood to the left ventricle and left atrium. The right coronary artery, which divides into the right posterior descending and acute marginal arteries, supply oxygenated blood to the right atrium and both the ventricles, sinoatrial node (cluster of cells in the right atrial wall that regulates the heart's rhythmic rate), and atrioventricular node.

Coronary veins

The coronary veins return deoxygenated blood (containing metabolic waste products) from the myocardium to the right atrium. This blood then flows back to the lungs for reoxygenation and removal of carbon dioxide.

Coronary veins contain valves preventing back flow; a Thebesian valve may or may not cover the ostium of the coronary sinus. Typically cardiac veins are free of atherosclerotic plaques. The coronary sinus is a collection of veins joined together to form a large vessel that collects blood from the heart muscle (myocardium) (Figure 16.3). It delivers deoxygenated blood to the right atrium.

The coronary sinus opens into the right atrium, at the coronary sinus orifice, between the inferior vena cava and the right atrioventricular orifice. It returns the blood from the substance of the heart, and is protected by a semi-circular fold of the lining membrane of the auricle.

17 The conducting system

Figure 17.1 Conducting system of the heart

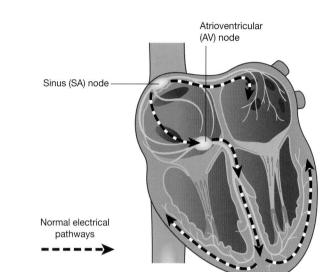

Atrioventricular
(AV) node

Sinus (SA) node

Normal electrical
pathways

Source:
Peate I, Wild K & Nair M (eds) Nursing Practice:
Knowledge and Care (2014)

Figure 17.2 Cardiac cycle

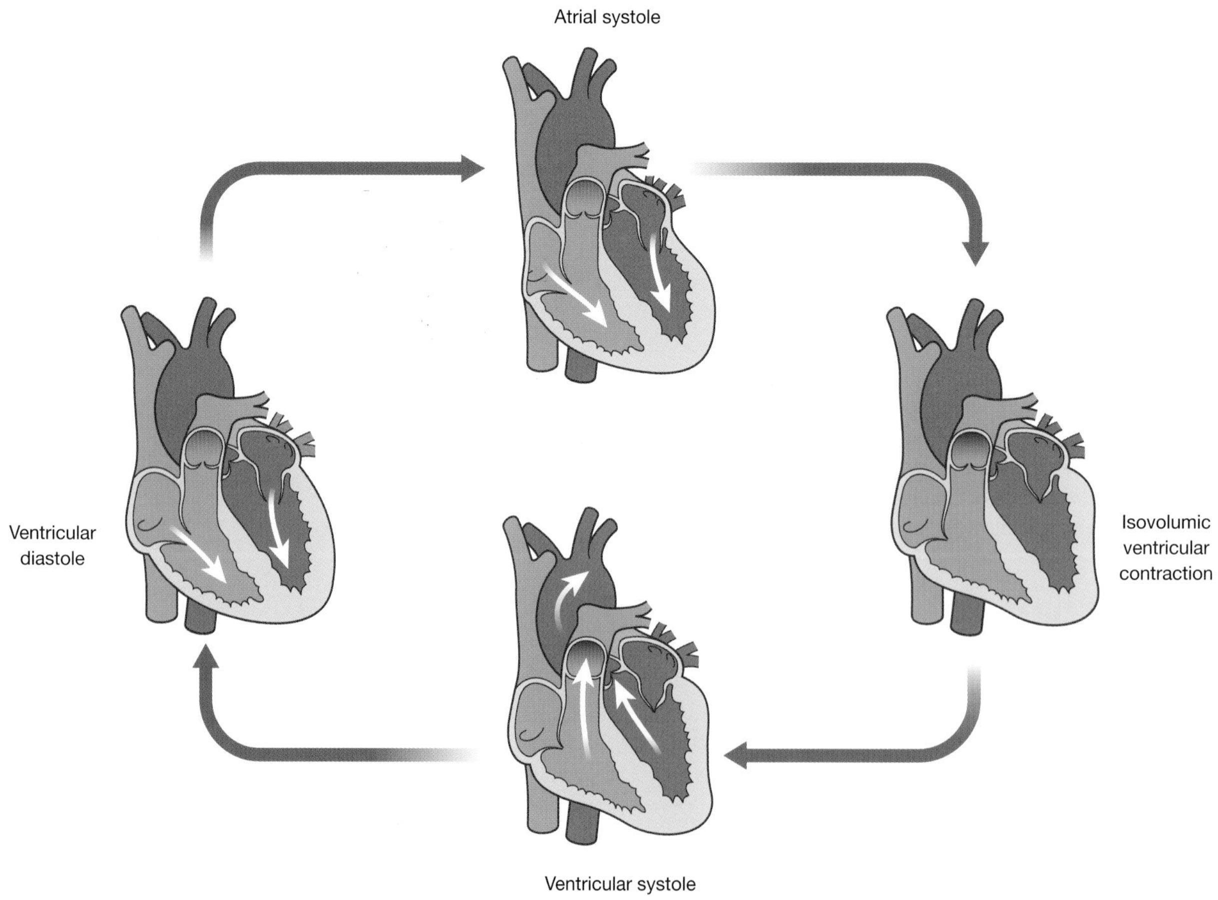

Atrial systole

Ventricular
diastole

Isovolumic
ventricular
contraction

Ventricular systole

Anatomy and Physiology for Nurses at a Glance, First Edition. Ian Peate and Muralitharan Nair. © 2015 John Wiley & Sons, Ltd. Published 2015 by John Wiley & Sons, Ltd.
Companion website: www.ataglanceseries.com/nursing/anatomy

Cardiac conduction

Cardiac conduction is the rate at which the heart conducts electrical impulses. These impulses cause the heart to contract and then relax. The constant cycle of heart muscle contraction followed by relaxation cause blood to be pumped throughout the body. The conduction pathway is made up of five elements (Figure 17.1):

1 the sino-atrial (SA) node,
2 the atrioventricular (AV) node,
3 the bundle of His,
4 the left and right bundle branches,
5 the Purkinje fibres.

SA node

The SA node is the natural pacemaker of the heart, which is located in the right atrium (Figure 17.1). The SA node is a spindle-shaped structure composed of a fibrous tissue matrix with closely packed cells. The SA node releases electrical stimuli at a regular rate. The rate is dictated by the needs of the body. Each stimulus passes through the myocardial cells of the atria creating a wave of contraction which spreads rapidly through both atria.

The heart is made up of around half a billion cells. The majority of the cells make up the ventricular walls. The rapidity of atrial contraction is such that around 100 million myocardial cells contract in less than one third of a second. So fast, that the contraction of the atria appears instantaneous.

AV node

The AV node lies on the right side of the partition that divides the atria, near the bottom of the right atrium (Figure 17.1). When the impulses from the SA node reach the AV node they are delayed for about a tenth of a second. This delay allows the atria to contract and empty their contents first. The AV node regulates the signals to the ventricles to prevent rapid conduction (atrial fibrillation), as well as making sure that the atria are empty and closed before stimulating the ventricles.

Bundle of His

The bundle of His is a collection of heart muscle cells specialised for electrical conduction that transmits the electrical impulses from the AV node to the point of the apex of the fascicular branches. This bundle is the only site where action potential can conduct from the atria to the ventricles.

Left and right bundle branches

This is a segment of the network of specialised conducting fibres that transmits electrical impulses within the ventricles of the heart. Bundle branches are a continuation of the atrioventricular (AV) bundle, which extends from the upper part of the intraventricular septum. The AV bundle divides into a left and a right branch, each going to its respective ventricle by passing down the septum and beneath the endocardium. Within the ventricles the bundle branches subdivide and terminate in the Purkinje fibres.

Purkinje fibres

These fibres are located in the inner ventricular walls of the heart. These fibres consist of specialised cardiomyocytes that are able to conduct cardiac action potentials more quickly and efficiently than any other cells in the heart (Figure 17.1). Purkinje fibres allow the heart's conduction system to create synchronised contractions of its ventricles, and are therefore essential for maintaining a consistent heart rhythm.

Cardiac cycle

The cardiac cycle is the sequence of events that occurs when the heart beats (Figure 17.2). There are two phases of the cardiac cycle. In the diastole phase, the heart ventricles are relaxed and the heart fills with blood. In the systole phase, the ventricles contract and pump blood to the arteries. One cardiac cycle is completed when the heart fills with blood and the blood is pumped out of the heart.

First diastole phase

During the diastole phase, the atria and ventricles are relaxed and the atrioventricular valves are open. Deoxygenated blood from the superior and inferior vena cavae flows into the right atrium. The open atrioventricular valves allow blood to pass through to the ventricles. The SA node contracts, triggering the atria to contract. The right atrium empties its contents into the right ventricle. The tricuspid valve prevents the blood from flowing back into the right atrium.

First systole phase

During the systole phase, the right ventricle receives impulses from the Purkinje fibres and contracts. The atrioventricular valves close and the semilunar valves open. The deoxygenated blood is pumped into the pulmonary artery. The pulmonary valve prevents the blood from flowing back into the right ventricle. The pulmonary artery carries the blood to the lungs for gas exchange. The oxygenated blood returns to the left atrium by the pulmonary veins.

Second diastole phase

In the next diastole period, the semilunar valves close and the atrioventricular valves open. Blood from the pulmonary veins fills the left atrium. (Blood from the venae cavae are also filling the right atrium.) The SA node contracts again triggering the atria to contract. The left atrium empties its contents into the left ventricle. The mitral valve prevents the oxygenated blood from flowing back into the left atrium.

Second systole phase

During the following systole phase, the atrioventricular valves close and the semilunar valves open. The left ventricle receives impulses from the Purkinje fibres and contracts. Oxygenated blood is pumped into the aorta. The aortic valve prevents the oxygenated blood from flowing back into the left ventricle. The aorta branches out to provide oxygenated blood to all parts of the body. The oxygen depleted blood is returned to the heart via the vena cavae.

18 Nerve supply to the heart

Figure 18.1 Cardioregulatory centre

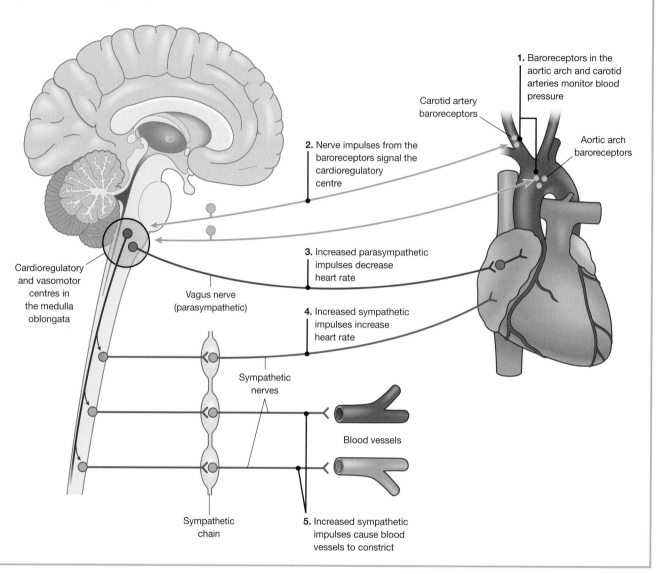

1. Baroreceptors in the aortic arch and carotid arteries monitor blood pressure

Carotid artery baroreceptors

Aortic arch baroreceptors

2. Nerve impulses from the baroreceptors signal the cardioregulatory centre

3. Increased parasympathetic impulses decrease heart rate

Cardioregulatory and vasomotor centres in the medulla oblongata

Vagus nerve (parasympathetic)

4. Increased sympathetic impulses increase heart rate

Sympathetic nerves

Blood vessels

Sympathetic chain

5. Increased sympathetic impulses cause blood vessels to constrict

Anatomy and Physiology for Nurses at a Glance, First Edition. Ian Peate and Muralitharan Nair. © 2015 John Wiley & Sons, Ltd. Published 2015 by John Wiley & Sons, Ltd.
Companion website: www.ataglanceseries.com/nursing/anatomy

Autonomic nervous system

Nervous system regulation of the heart originates in the cardioregulatory centre in the medulla oblongata (Figure 18.1). This region of the brain stem receives input from a variety of sensory receptors and from higher brain centres such as the limbic system and the cerebral cortex.

When activated by a stimulus, such as exercise or stress, the sympathetic nerve fibres release norepinephrine at their cardiac endings as a neurotransmitter. This leads to the excitation of the sinoatrial node and an increase in its production of action potentials and thus an increase in heart rate.

Alternatively when the parasympathetic nervous system is stimulated this results in the release of acetylcholine at the parasympathetic cardiac nerve endings, which has the effect of reducing the rate of action potential generation in the sinoatrial node and thus reducing heart rate.

Both the sympathetic and parasympathetic nervous systems are active at all times but the parasympathetic nervous system normally has the dominant influence. This can be seen if the vagus nerve (cranial nerve X) is cut, for instance in heart transplant patients. In these situations the sinoatrial node will normally produce action potentials at a rate of 100 a minute and therefore the heart rate increases to 100 beats per minute. The removal of the influence of the parasympathetic nervous system (by the disconnection of the vagus nerves) removes the heart rate reducing effect of this system.

The right vagus nerve primarily innervates the SA node, whereas the left vagus innervates the AV node; however, significant overlap can exist in the anatomical distribution.

Chemical regulation of the heart

Certain chemicals influence the heart rate. Hypoxia, acidosis and alkalosis all depress cardiac activity.

Hormones

Epinephrine and norepinephrine from the adrenal gland increase the heart rate and contractility. Stress, physical activity and excitement stimulate the adrenal gland to secrete more hormones, increasing the activity of the heart. Thyroid hormones from the thyroid gland also increase the heart rate and contractility. These hormones affect cardiac muscle fibres in much the same way as norepinephrine by the sympathetic nervous system; they increase both heart rate and contractility.

Ions

The difference in the levels of cations between the intracellular and extracellular fluid are important for the production of action potentials in all nerve and muscle fibres. For example, the concentration of potassium, sodium and calcium have a large effect on cardiac function. An elevated level of potassium or sodium can decrease the heart rate and contractility. An increase in intracellular calcium levels increases heart rate and strengthens the heart beat. On the other hand, excess sodium blocks calcium entry into the cells thus decreasing the force of contraction and excess potassium blocks action potentials.

Baroreceptors

Baroreceptors are specialised mechanical receptors located in the carotid sinus and the aortic arch. They are sensitive to the amount of stretch in these blood vessels and have direct outflow via the autonomic nervous system to the cardiovascular centre in the medulla oblongata.

The cardiovascular centre of the medulla oblongata is the main centre for the control of autonomic nervous activity that affects the heart. The cardiovascular centre is made up of two sub-centres:

Cardioinhibitory centre

This centre directly controls parasympathetic outflow to the heart (especially the sinoatrial node), thus increased outflow from this centre has the effect of reducing heart rate. The neurotransmitter, acetylcholine, directly stimulates the heart to decrease cardiac output to return the circulatory system to a resting homeostasis after the end of episodes of increased muscular activity or fight-or-flight emergencies; this centre plays the more minor role in controlling cardiac output.

Vasomotor centre

This is further divided into the pressor area and the depressor area. The pressor area has a relatively constant outflow of action potentials to the heart via the sympathetic nervous system. This has a direct effect on both heart rate and the force of ventricular contraction (and therefore stroke volume) as well as effects on the vasculature which subsequently will affect heart function by changing preload and afterload. Outflow from the pressor area is moderated by nerves transmitting impulses from the depressor area which have a directly inhibiting effect on the transmission of impulses from the pressor area. Thus it can be thought of that the nerve impulses of the depressor area act like a 'collar' or tap; the greater the number of impulses from the depressor area the tighter the collar or tap is made, reducing the number of impulses from the pressor area to the heart and thus the effect on heart rate and force of contraction.

Other factors in heart regulation

Other factors that can affect heart rate include exercise, gender, body temperature and age.

Body temperature

Temperature affects several processes inside the body. When body temperature goes up, blood vessels dilate which increases heart rate, in order to compensate for drop in blood pressure. On the other hand, a decrease in temperature can lower the heart rate but only to some degree. If the temperature gets too low, the body will actually increase the heart rate, while trying to warm up.

Body fluid level

Dehydration decreases the amount of fluids in the blood which causes constriction of coronary arteries. At the same time, the heart begins to beat faster, in order to push the thicker blood through the blood vessels.

19 Structure of the blood vessels

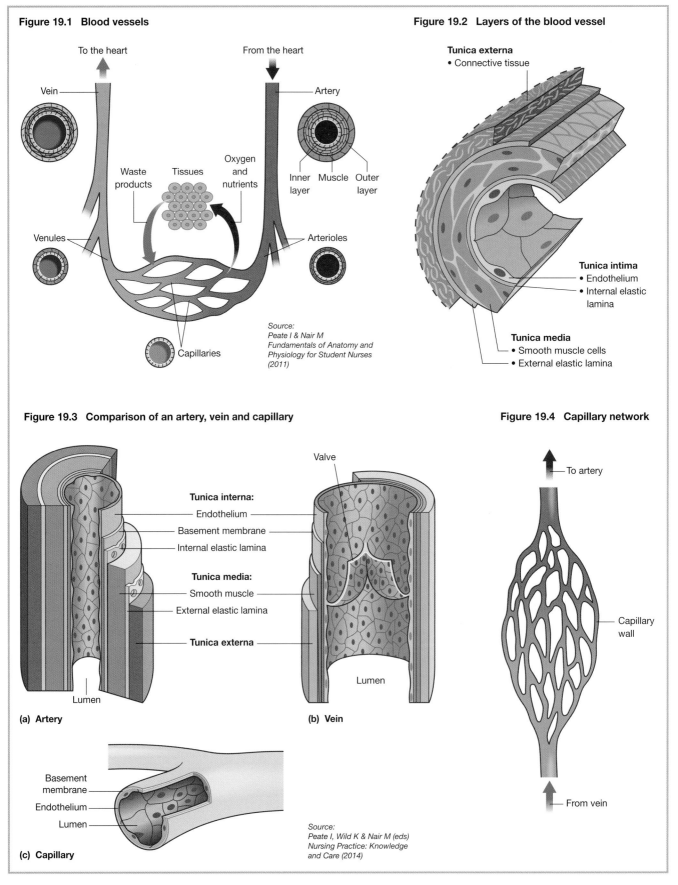

Figure 19.1 Blood vessels

To the heart

From the heart

Vein

Artery

Waste products

Tissues

Oxygen and nutrients

Inner layer   Muscle   Outer layer

Venules

Arterioles

Capillaries

Source:
Peate I & Nair M
Fundamentals of Anatomy and
Physiology for Student Nurses
(2011)

Figure 19.2 Layers of the blood vessel

Tunica externa
• Connective tissue

Tunica intima
• Endothelium
• Internal elastic lamina

Tunica media
• Smooth muscle cells
• External elastic lamina

Figure 19.3 Comparison of an artery, vein and capillary

Valve

Tunica interna:
— Endothelium
— Basement membrane
— Internal elastic lamina

Tunica media:
— Smooth muscle
— External elastic lamina

Tunica externa

Lumen

Lumen

(a) Artery

(b) Vein

Basement membrane

Endothelium

Lumen

(c) Capillary

Source:
Peate I, Wild K & Nair M (eds)
Nursing Practice: Knowledge
and Care (2014)

Figure 19.4 Capillary network

To artery

Capillary wall

From vein

Blood vessels

Blood vessels are part of the circulatory system that transports blood throughout the body. There are three major types of blood vessels: the arteries, which carry the blood away from the heart; the capillaries, which enable the actual exchange of water, nutrients and chemicals between the blood and the tissues; and the veins, which carry blood from the capillaries back towards the heart (Figure 19.1). All arteries, with the exception of the pulmonary and umbilical arteries, carry oxygenated blood, while most veins carry deoxygenated blood from the tissues back to the heart; with the exceptions of pulmonary and umbilical veins, both of which carry oxygenated blood. The capillaries form the microcirculatory system and it is at this point that nutrients, gases, water and electrolytes are exchanged between the blood and the tissue fluid. Capillaries are tiny, extremely thin-walled vessels that act as a bridge between arteries and veins. The thin walls of the capillaries allow oxygen and nutrients to pass from the blood into tissue fluid and allow waste products to pass from tissue fluid into the blood.

Structure

The walls of the larger blood vessels consist of three layers: tunica intima consisting of thin layer of endothelial cells, tunic media containing smooth muscles and elastic fibres and an outer layer called tunica externa consisting of fibroblasts, nerves and collagenous tissue (Figure 19.2). The endothelium is an epithelial lining that is only one-cell-thick. Therefore, the tunica interna is always very, very thin.

Arteries

Arteries receive blood under high pressure from the ventricles of the heart. They must therefore be able to stretch each time the heart beats, without collapsing under the increased pressure. The walls of arteries consist of three layers, namely an outer layer, a thick middle layer and an inner layer. The outer layer consists of white fibrous connective tissue which merges to the outside with the loose connective tissue in which artery is found (Figure 19.3). This helps to anchor the arteries because the heart pumps the blood through the arteries at a great pressure. The thick middle layer consists of elastic connective tissue and involuntary muscle tissue. This layer is supplied with two sets of nerves, one stimulating the muscles to relax so that the artery is allowed to widen, and the other one causing the circular muscles to contract, making the artery become narrower. The inner layer of endothelium consists of flat epithelial cells which are packed closely together and which is continuous with the endocardium of the heart. The flat cells make the inside lining of the arteries smooth to limit friction between the blood and the lining to a minimum.

Veins

Since veins carry blood back to the heart, the pressure exerted by the heart beat on them is much less than in the arteries. The middle muscular wall of a vein is therefore much thinner than that of an artery. Veins differ from arteries also in that they have semi-lunar valves, which prevent the blood from flowing backwards (Figure 19.3). The vein valves are necessary to keep blood flowing toward the heart, but they are also necessary to allow blood to flow against the force of gravity. For example, blood that is returning to the heart from the foot has to be able to flow up the leg. Generally, the force of gravity would discourage that from happening. The vein valves, however, provide footholds for the blood as it flows its way up. The valves are like gates that only allow traffic to move in one direction.

Veins receive blood from the capillaries after the exchange of oxygen and carbon dioxide has taken place. Therefore, the veins transport carbon dioxide rich blood back to the lungs and heart. It is important that the carbon dioxide rich blood keeps moving in the proper direction and not be allowed to flow backward; this is accomplished by valves that are in the veins.

Capillaries

Capillaries are tiny blood vessels, of approximately 5–20 micrometres diameter. There are networks of capillaries (Figure 19.4) in most of the organs and tissues of the body. Capillary walls are only one cell thick, which allows exchanges of material between the contents of the capillary and the surrounding tissue fluid. The walls of capillaries are composed of only a single layer of cells, the endothelium (Figure 19.3). This layer is so thin that molecules such as oxygen, water and lipids can pass through them by diffusion and enter the tissues. Waste products such as carbon dioxide and urea can diffuse back into the blood to be carried away for removal from the body. Capillaries are so small the red blood cells need to change its shapes in order to pass through them in single file.

The flow of blood in the capillaries is controlled by structures called precapillary sphincters. These structures are located between arterioles and capillaries and contain muscle fibres that allow them to contract. When the sphincters are open, blood flows freely to the capillary beds of body tissue. When the sphincters are closed, blood is not allowed to flow through the capillary beds. Fluid exchange between the capillaries and the body tissues takes place at the capillary bed.

20 Blood pressure

Figure 20.1 Baroreceptors

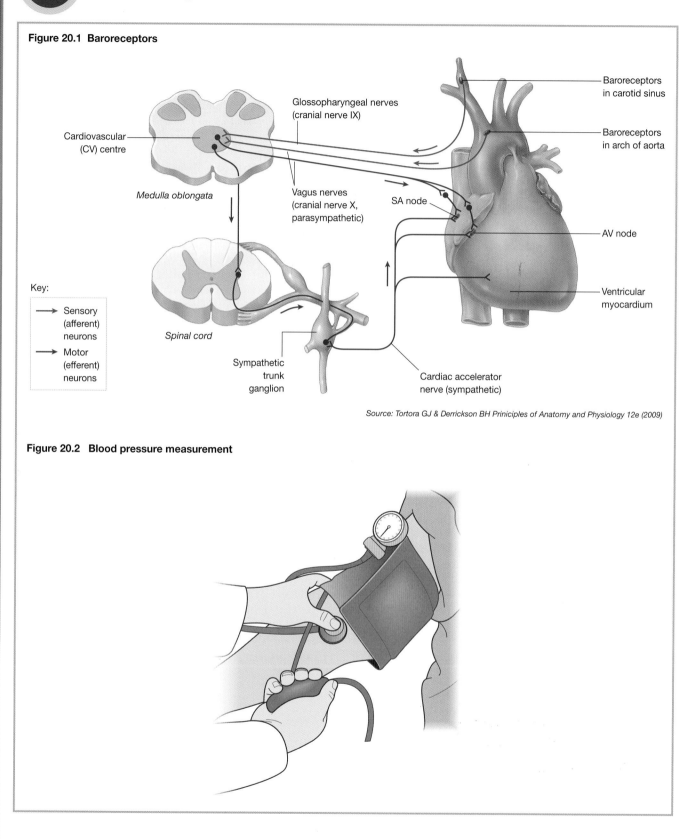

Glossopharyngeal nerves
(cranial nerve IX)

Cardiovascular
(CV) centre

Medulla oblongata

Vagus nerves
(cranial nerve X,
parasympathetic)

SA node

Baroreceptors
in carotid sinus

Baroreceptors
in arch of aorta

AV node

Ventricular
myocardium

Key:

→ Sensory
(afferent)
neurons

→ Motor
(efferent)
neurons

Spinal cord

Sympathetic
trunk
ganglion

Cardiac accelerator
nerve (sympathetic)

Source: Tortora GJ & Derrickson BH Priniciples of Anatomy and Physiology 12e (2009)

Figure 20.2 Blood pressure measurement

Anatomy and Physiology for Nurses at a Glance, First Edition. Ian Peate and Muralitharan Nair. © 2015 John Wiley & Sons, Ltd. Published 2015 by John Wiley & Sons, Ltd.
Companion website: www.ataglanceseries.com/nursing/anatomy

What is blood pressure?

Blood pressure is the pressure exerted by blood within the blood vessel. The pressure is at its greatest nearer the heart but decreases as the blood moves away from the heart. Three factors regulate blood pressure and they include: neuronal regulation – through the autonomic nervous system; hormonal regulation – adrenaline, noradrenaline, renin and others; and auto-regulation – through the renin-angiotensin system

Physiological factors

Many factors influence arterial blood pressure, which may be affected by other factors such as age, gender, hormones, disease and exercise. The volume of blood that is present in the body affects blood pressure. An increase in blood volume in the body increases the rate of blood flow to the heart resulting in increased cardiac output.

Peripheral resistance is another physiological factor. In the circulatory system, this is the resistance of the blood vessels. The higher the resistance, the higher the arterial pressure upstream from the resistance to blood flow. Resistance is related to vessel radius (the larger the radius, the lower the resistance), vessel length (the longer the vessel, the higher the resistance), blood viscosity, as well as the smoothness of the blood vessel walls. An increase in viscosity of the blood increases blood pressure. The resistance is provided by plasma proteins and other substances in the blood.

The blood pressure changes in response to changes in cardiac output. In other words, as the cardiac output increases, so does the blood pressure. If the cardiac output decreases, so does the blood pressure. If either the stroke volume or the heart rate increases, so does the cardiac output and, as a result, the blood pressure rises. Conversely, if the stroke volume or the heart rate decreases, so do both the cardiac output and the blood pressure. The volume of blood pumped out from the ventricle with each contraction is called the stroke volume and equals about 70 ml for an adult at rest.

Control of blood pressure

This is regulated by many factors, such as baroreceptors, chemoreceptors, hypothalamus, circulating hormones and the renin-angiotensin system.

Baroreceptors

These are situated in the arch of the aorta and the carotid sinus and they are sensitive to pressure changes within the blood vessel. When the blood pressure increases, signals are sent to cardio-regulatory centre (CRC) in the brain stem (medulla oblongata) (Figure 20.1). The cardio-regulatory centre increases the parasympathetic activity to the heart, reducing heart rate and inhibiting sympathetic activity to the blood vessels, causing vasodilatation. This reduces blood pressure. On the other hand, if the blood pressure falls, the CRC increases the sympathetic activity to the heart and the blood vessels thus increasing heart rate and vasoconstriction resulting in increased blood pressure.

Chemoreceptors

Chemoreceptors are found close to the carotid and aortic baroreceptors in small structures called carotid bodies and aortic bodies. They are sensitive to any change in the chemical composition of the blood, such as a decrease in oxygen level and pH of the blood or an increase in the carbon dioxide level. These receptors send impulses to the cardiovascular centre which in turn increase the sympathetic stimulation to the blood vessels causing an increase in blood pressure. Chemoreceptors also stimulate the respiratory centres in the brain to increase the rate of respiration.

Circulating hormones

Hormones such as anti-diuretic (ADH) and atrial natriuretic peptide (ANP) help to regulate circulating blood volume by fluid and electrolyte regulation, thus affecting blood pressure. It is released when the body is dehydrated and causes the kidneys to conserve water, thus concentrating the urine and reducing its volume. At high concentrations, it also raises blood pressure by inducing moderate vasoconstriction.

ANP is a powerful vasodilator, and a protein (polypeptide) hormone secreted by heart muscle cells. It is released by the atria of the heart. ANP acts to reduce the water, sodium and adipose levels in the circulatory system, thereby reducing blood pressure.

Renin-angiotensin system

This help to maintain blood pressure though its action on vasoconstriction by generating angiotensin II (Figure 19.2). When blood volume is low, juxtaglomerular cells in the kidneys secrete renin directly into circulation. Plasma renin then carries out the conversion of angiotensinogen released by the liver to angiotensin I. Angiotensin I is subsequently converted to angiotensin II by the angiotensin converting enzyme found in the lungs. Angiotensin II is a potent vaso-active peptide that causes blood vessels to constrict, resulting in increased blood pressure.

Angiotensin II stimulates the release of the hormone aldosterone in the adrenal glands, which causes the renal tubules to retain sodium and water and excrete potassium. Together, angiotensin II and aldosterone work to raise blood volume, blood pressure and sodium levels in the blood to restore the balance of sodium, potassium and fluids. If the renin-angiotensin system becomes overactive, consistently high blood pressure results.

Hypothalamus

The hypothalamus responds to stimuli such as emotion, pain and anger, and stimulates sympathetic nervous activity affecting blood pressure.

Taking blood pressure

Blood pressure is measured using a sphygmomanometer (electronic, digital or aneroids) and it is a non-invasive method of monitoring a patient's blood pressure (Figure 20.2). It may be used as a diagnostic test on patients with arterial blood pressure problems. It can be recorded with the patient sitting comfortably in a chair or lying in bed. Taking and recording blood pressure is a skill that all nurses need to be competent in.

Ambulatory blood pressure monitoring is also sometimes used to check how well medicine used to treat hypertension is working.

21 Lymphatic circulation

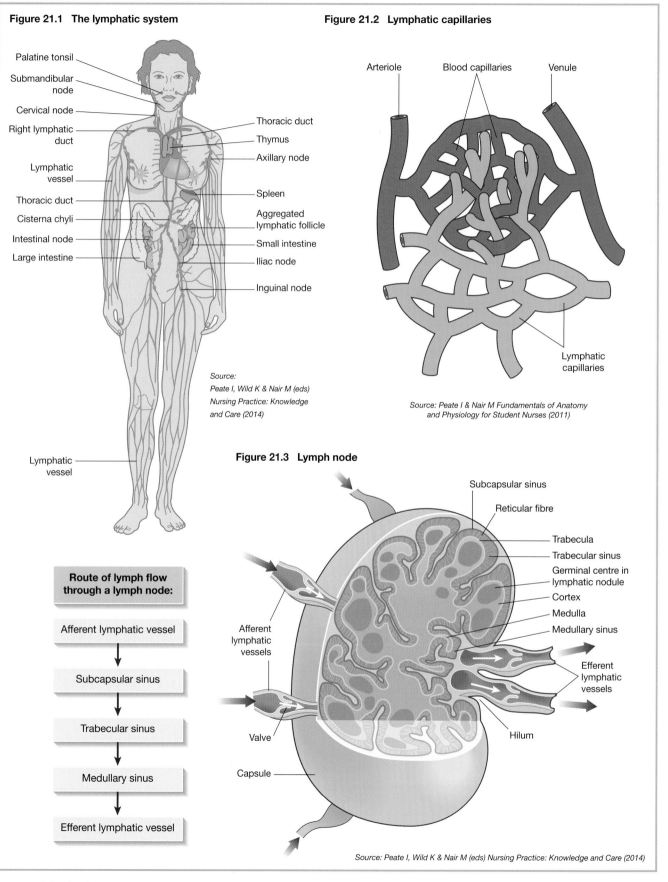

Figure 21.1 The lymphatic system

- Palatine tonsil
- Submandibular node
- Cervical node
- Right lymphatic duct
- Lymphatic vessel
- Thoracic duct
- Cisterna chyli
- Intestinal node
- Large intestine
- Thoracic duct
- Thymus
- Axillary node
- Spleen
- Aggregated lymphatic follicle
- Small intestine
- Iliac node
- Inguinal node
- Lymphatic vessel

Source:
Peate I, Wild K & Nair M (eds)
Nursing Practice: Knowledge
and Care (2014)

Figure 21.2 Lymphatic capillaries

- Arteriole
- Blood capillaries
- Venule
- Lymphatic capillaries

Source: Peate I & Nair M Fundamentals of Anatomy
and Physiology for Student Nurses (2011)

Figure 21.3 Lymph node

- Subcapsular sinus
- Reticular fibre
- Trabecula
- Trabecular sinus
- Germinal centre in lymphatic nodule
- Cortex
- Medulla
- Medullary sinus
- Efferent lymphatic vessels
- Hilum
- Afferent lymphatic vessels
- Valve
- Capsule

Route of lymph flow through a lymph node:

Afferent lymphatic vessel
↓
Subcapsular sinus
↓
Trabecular sinus
↓
Medullary sinus
↓
Efferent lymphatic vessel

Source: Peate I, Wild K & Nair M (eds) Nursing Practice: Knowledge and Care (2014)

Anatomy and Physiology for Nurses at a Glance, First Edition. Ian Peate and Muralitharan Nair. © 2015 John Wiley & Sons, Ltd. Published 2015 by John Wiley & Sons, Ltd.
Companion website: www.ataglanceseries.com/nursing/anatomy

Lymphatic system

The lymphatic system is a network of tissues and organs that primarily consists of lymph vessels, lymph nodes and lymph. The tonsils, adenoids, spleen and thymus are all part of the lymphatic system (Figure 21.1). There are 600 to 700 lymph nodes in the human body that filter the lymph before it returns to the circulatory system.

The spleen, which is largest lymphatic organ, is located on the left side of the body just above the kidney. Humans can live without a spleen, although people who have lost their spleen to disease or injury are more prone to infections.

The thymus, which stores immature lymphocytes and prepares them to become active T cells, is located in the chest just above the heart.

Tonsils are large clusters of lymphatic cells found in the pharynx. Although tonsillectomies occur much less frequently today than they did in the 1950s, it is still among the most common operations performed and typically follows frequent throat infections.

Lymphatic capillaries (Figure 21.2) differ from blood capillaries in that they originate as pockets rather than forming continuous vessels, have larger diameters, thinner walls and have an irregular outline.

What is lymph?

Lymph is a clear fluid found inside the lymphatic capillaries and it has a similar composition to plasma. Lymph is the ultra-filtrate of the blood which occurs at the capillary ends of the blood vessels.

This fluid contains white blood cells, known as lymphocytes, along with a small concentration of red blood cells and proteins. It circulates freely through the body, bathing cells in needed nutrients and oxygen while it collects harmful materials for disposal. Lymph may pick up bacteria and bring them to lymph nodes where they are destroyed.

Lymph nodes

Lymph nodes are bean shaped organs scattered along the lymphatic vessels. These nodes are found in the largest concentrations at the neck, armpit, thorax, abdomen and the groin (Figure 20.3) and lesser concentrations are found behind the elbows and knees.

Lymph vessels route the fluid through nodes that are located throughout the body. Lymph nodes are small structures that work as filters for harmful substances. They contain immune cells that can attack and destroy germs in the lymph fluid to help fight infection. Each lymph node filters fluid and substances picked up by the vessels that lead to it. Lymph fluid from the fingers, for instance, works its way toward the chest, joining fluid from the arm. This fluid may filter through lymph nodes at the elbow, or those under the arm. Fluid from the head, scalp and face flows down through lymph nodes in the neck. At the end of the circulation useful substances such as protein and salts are returned to the general circulation.

Lymphatic organs
Spleen

The spleen (Figure 21.1) is an organ about the size of a clenched fist found on the left-hand side of the upper abdomen. Its main functions are to filter your blood, create new blood cells and store platelets. It is also a key part of your body's immune system.

The spleen contains two main types of tissue: white pulp and red pulp. White pulp is lymphatic tissue (material which is part of the immune system) mainly made up of white blood cells. Red pulp is made up of venous sinuses (blood-filled cavities) and splenic cords. Splenic cords are special tissues which contain different types of red and white blood cells.

Blood flows into the spleen where it enters the white pulp. Here, white blood cells called B and T cells screen the blood flowing through. T cells help to recognise invading pathogens (germs – for example, bacteria and viruses) that might cause illness and then destroy them. B cells make antibodies that help to stop infections from spreading.

Blood also enters the red pulp where the damaged red blood cells are removed and stores platelets. In unborn babies red pulp produces new red blood cells; however this function stops after birth.

Thymus gland

The thymus (Figure 21.1) is of a pinkish-grey colour, soft and lobulated on its surfaces. At birth it is about 5 cm in length, 4 cm in breadth and about 6 mm in thickness. The thymus is an important part of children's immune systems. It grows larger until puberty and then begins to shrink. The thymus gland consists of two lobes joined by a connective tissue and each lobe is covered by an outer cortex and an inner portion called the medulla.

The gland produces thymosins, which are hormones that stimulate the development of antibodies. The thymus also produces T-lymphocytes which are white blood cells that fight infections and destroy abnormal cells. Once matured, these T lymphocytes, or T cells, circulate through the bloodstream and collect in the lymph organs – the spleen and lymph nodes – for future use.

Functions of the lymphatic system

The lymphatic system destroys pathogens and filters waste, dead blood cells, pathogens, cancer cells and toxins before returning useful substances to the circulation. It delivers oxygen, nutrients and hormones from the blood to the cells.

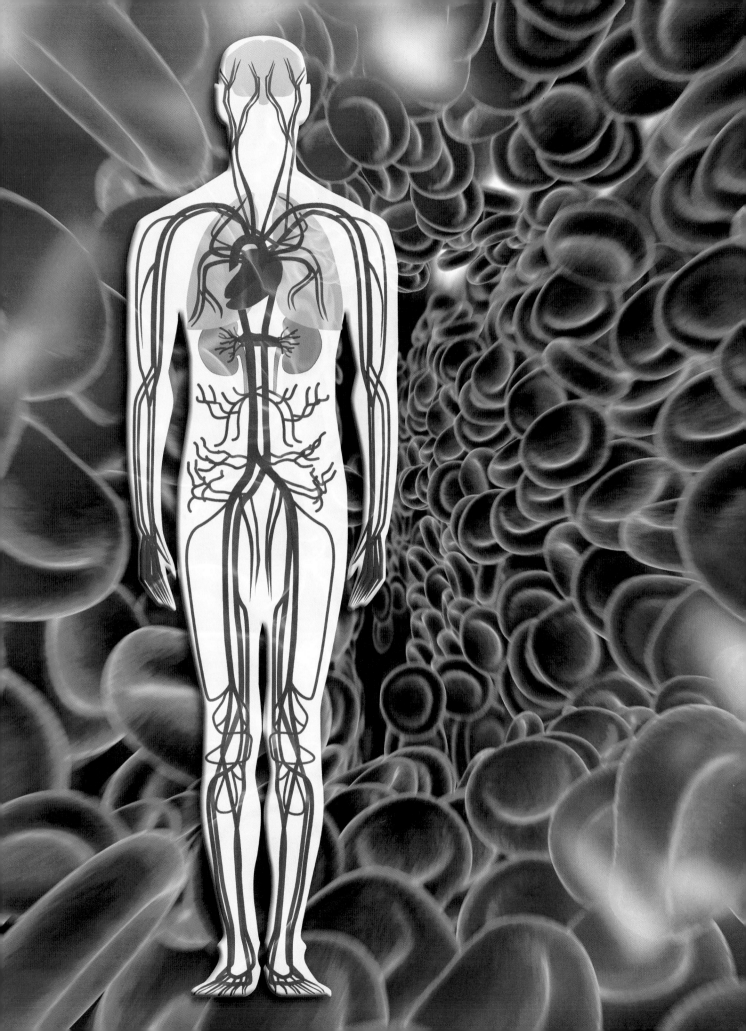

The respiratory system

Part 4

Chapters

22 The respiratory tract

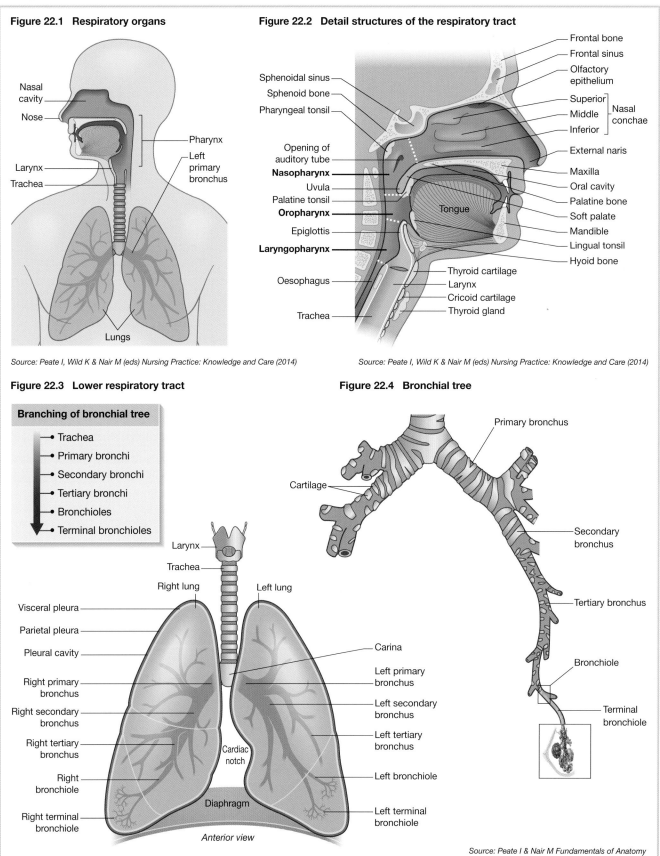

Figure 22.1 Respiratory organs

- Nasal cavity
- Nose
- Pharynx
- Larynx
- Left primary bronchus
- Trachea
- Lungs

Source: Peate I, Wild K & Nair M (eds) Nursing Practice: Knowledge and Care (2014)

Figure 22.2 Detail structures of the respiratory tract

- Sphenoidal sinus
- Sphenoid bone
- Pharyngeal tonsil
- Opening of auditory tube
- **Nasopharynx**
- Uvula
- Palatine tonsil
- **Oropharynx**
- Epiglottis
- **Laryngopharynx**
- Oesophagus
- Trachea
- Frontal bone
- Frontal sinus
- Olfactory epithelium
- Superior
- Middle — Nasal conchae
- Inferior
- External naris
- Maxilla
- Oral cavity
- Palatine bone
- Soft palate
- Mandible
- Lingual tonsil
- Hyoid bone
- Thyroid cartilage
- Larynx
- Cricoid cartilage
- Thyroid gland
- Tongue

Source: Peate I, Wild K & Nair M (eds) Nursing Practice: Knowledge and Care (2014)

Figure 22.3 Lower respiratory tract

Branching of bronchial tree
- Trachea
- Primary bronchi
- Secondary bronchi
- Tertiary bronchi
- Bronchioles
- Terminal bronchioles

- Larynx
- Trachea
- Right lung
- Left lung
- Visceral pleura
- Parietal pleura
- Pleural cavity
- Right primary bronchus
- Right secondary bronchus
- Right tertiary bronchus
- Right bronchiole
- Right terminal bronchiole
- Cardiac notch
- Diaphragm
- Carina
- Left primary bronchus
- Left secondary bronchus
- Left tertiary bronchus
- Left bronchiole
- Left terminal bronchiole

Anterior view

Source: Peate I, Wild K & Nair M (eds) Nursing Practice: Knowledge and Care (2014)

Figure 22.4 Bronchial tree

- Primary bronchus
- Cartilage
- Secondary bronchus
- Tertiary bronchus
- Bronchiole
- Terminal bronchiole

Source: Peate I & Nair M Fundamentals of Anatomy and Physiology for Student Nurses (2011)

Anatomy and Physiology for Nurses at a Glance, First Edition. Ian Peate and Muralitharan Nair. © 2015 John Wiley & Sons, Ltd. Published 2015 by John Wiley & Sons, Ltd.
Companion website: www.ataglanceseries.com/nursing/anatomy

Respiratory system

The respiratory system is responsible for gaseous exchange between the circulatory system and the atmosphere. Air is taken in via the upper airways (the nasal cavity, pharynx and larynx) through the lower airways (trachea, primary bronchi and bronchial tree) and into the small bronchioles and alveoli within the lung tissue (Figure 22.1).

Upper respiratory tract

Mouth, nose, nasal cavity and pharynx are the organs of the upper respiratory tract. The functions of this part of the system are to warm, filter and moisten the inhaled air. The nasal cavity is divided into two equal sections by the nasal septum, a structure formed out of the ethmoid bones and the vomer of the skull. The space where air enters the nasal cavity just inside the nostrils is referred to as the vestibule.

The nasal cavities are subdivided into three air passageways, the meatuses, which are formed by three shelf-like projections called the superior, middle and inferior conchae or turbinates. The incoming air bounces off the conchal surface and swirls. Small particles in the air are then trapped in the mucosa of the nasal cavity (Figure 22.2).

The pharynx is a chamber shared by the digestive and respiratory systems. The pharynx connects the nasal and oral cavity with the larynx. The pharynx is divided into three regions called the nasopharynx, the oropharynx and the laryngopharynx. The nasopharynx sits behind the nasal cavity and contains two openings that lead to the auditory (Eustachian) tubes.

Both the oropharynx and the laryngopharynx are passageways for food and drink as well as air and they are lined with non-keratinised stratified squamous epithelium.

Lower respiratory tract

The lower respiratory tract includes the larynx, the trachea, the right and left primary bronchi and all the constituents of both lungs (Figure 22.3). The lungs are two coned-shaped organs that almost fill the thorax. They are protected by a framework of bones, the thoracic cage, which consists of the ribs, sternum (breast bone) and vertebrae (spine). The air passages are lined with mucous membrane composed mainly of ciliated epithelium. Cilia constantly clean the tract and carry foreign matter upwards for swallowing or expectoration.

Larynx

The larynx consists of nine pieces of cartilage tissue, three single pieces and three pairs. The single pieces of cartilage are the thyroid, epiglottis and cricoid cartilage. The thyroid cartilage is more commonly known as the Adam's apple and together with the cricoid cartilage protects the vocal cords. The epiglottis is a leaf-shaped piece of elastic cartilage attached to the top of the larynx. Its function is to protect the airway from food and water. On swallowing, the epiglottis blocks entry to the larynx and food and liquids are diverted towards the oesophagus, which sits nearby.

Trachea

The trachea (windpipe) extends from the laryngopharynx at the level of the cricoid cartilage at the top to the carina (also called the tracheal bifurcation). The trachea contains 15–20 C-shaped cartilage rings that reinforce and protect the trachea to prevent it from collapsing or overexpansion as pressure changes within the respiratory system. The carina is a ridge-shaped structure at the level of T6 or T7. The carina possesses sensory nerve endings which cause coughing if food or water is inhaled accidently.

Bronchi and bronchioles

The human trachea (windpipe) divides into two main bronchi (also main stem bronchi), the left and the right, at the level of the sternal angle and of the fifth thoracic vertebra or up to two vertebrae higher or lower, depending on breathing, at the anatomical point known as the carina.

The right main bronchus is more vertical, wider and shorter, and subdivides into three lobar bronchi, the left main bronchus, which divides into two. The segmental bronchi divide into many primary bronchioles which divide into terminal bronchioles, each of which then gives rise to several respiratory bronchioles, which go on to divide into and terminate in tiny air sacs called alveoli (Figure 22.4).

Lungs

The lungs are divided into distinct regions called lobes. There are three lobes in the right lung and two in the left. Each lung is surrounded by two thin protective membranes called the parietal and visceral pleura. The parietal pleura line the wall of the thorax whereas the visceral pleura line the lungs themselves. The space between the two pleura, the pleural space, is minute and contains a thin film of lubricating fluid. This reduces friction between the two pleura, allowing both layers to slide over one another during breathing. The fluid also helps the visceral and parietal pleura to adhere to each other.

Blood supply

The conduction and respiratory regions of the lungs receive blood from different arteries. The conduction region of the lungs receives oxygenated blood from capillaries that stem from the bronchial arteries, which originate from the aorta. Some of the bronchial arteries are connected to the pulmonary arteries but the majority of blood returns to the heart via the pulmonary or bronchial veins.

Pulmonary ventilation

Figure 23.1 Boyle's Law

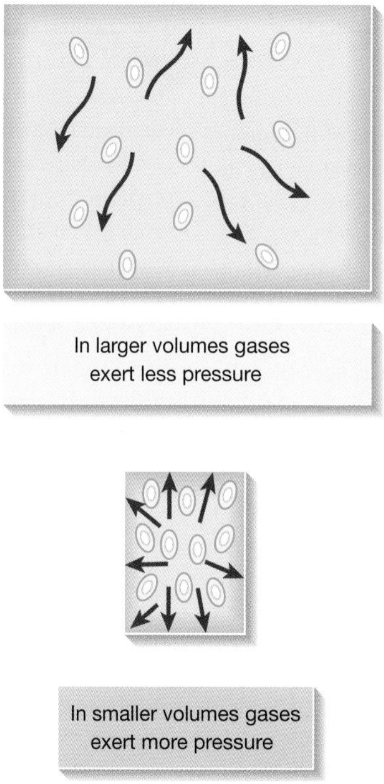

In larger volumes gases exert less pressure

In smaller volumes gases exert more pressure

Source: Peate I & Nair M Fundamentals of Anatomy and Physiology for Student Nurses (2011)

Figure 23.2 Inspiration and expiration

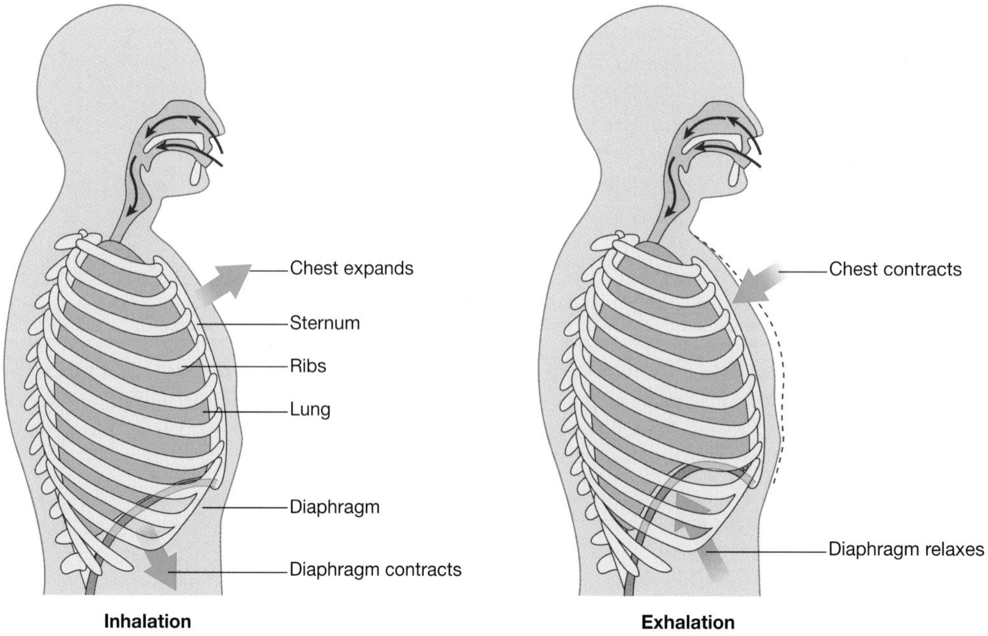

Chest expands

Sternum

Ribs

Lung

Diaphragm

Diaphragm contracts

Inhalation

Chest contracts

Diaphragm relaxes

Exhalation

Source: Peate I & Nair M Fundamentals of Anatomy and Physiology for Student Nurses (2011)

Anatomy and Physiology for Nurses at a Glance, First Edition. Ian Peate and Muralitharan Nair. © 2015 John Wiley & Sons, Ltd. Published 2015 by John Wiley & Sons, Ltd.
Companion website: www.ataglanceseries.com/nursing/anatomy

Breathing

Pulmonary ventilation involves physical movement of air in and out of lungs. The primary function of pulmonary ventilation is to maintain adequate alveolar ventilation. This prevents the build-up of carbon dioxide in the alveoli and achieves a constant supply of oxygen to the tissues.

Air flows between the atmosphere and the alveoli of the lungs as a result of pressure difference created by the contraction and relaxation of the respiratory muscles. The rate of air flow and the effort needed for breathing is influenced by the alveoli surface tension and integrity of the lungs.

Inspiration

Breathing is called inhalation. Just before breathing (inhalation) the pressure in the lungs equals the atmospheric pressure (760 mmHg or 101.33 kilopascals (kPa)). Thus for air to flow into the lungs, the pressure inside the alveoli must be lower than the atmosphere. This is achieved by increasing the volume of the lungs.

During inspiration the thorax expands and intrapulmonary pressure falls below atmospheric pressure. Because intrapulmonary pressure is now less than atmospheric pressure, air will naturally enter our lungs until the pressure difference no longer exists. This phenomenon is explained by Boyle's Law (Figure 23.1) and Dalton's Law. Gases exert pressure and Boyle's Law states that the amount of pressure exerted is inversely proportional to the size of its container.

Dalton's Law states that in a mixture of gases each gas exerts its own individual pressure that is proportional to its size. For example atmospheric air contains a mixture of gases. Each individual gas will exert its own pressure dependent upon its quantity. Nitrogen, for example, will exert the greatest pressure as it is the most abundant gas. Collectively all the gases in the atmosphere exert a pressure, atmospheric pressure, which is 101.33 kPa at sea level. On inhalation the thorax expands and intrapulmonary pressure falls below 101.33 kPa and air enters the lungs.

A range of respiratory muscles are used to achieve thoracic expansion during inspiration. The major muscles of inspiration are the diaphragm and external intercostal muscles. The diaphragm is a dome-shaped skeletal muscle found beneath the lungs at the base of the thorax. There are 11 external intercostal muscles, which sit in the intercostal spaces – the spaces between the ribs. During inspiration the diaphragm contracts downwards, pulling the lungs with it (Figure 23.2). Simultaneously the external intercostal muscles pull the rib cage outwards and upwards. The thorax is now bigger than before and intrapulmonary pressure is reduced below atmospheric pressure as a result. The most important muscle of inspiration is the diaphragm, 75% of the air that enters the lungs is as a result of diaphragmatic contraction.

Exhalation

Breathing out (exhalation) is also as a result of pressure gradient but it is converse to inhalation, that is the pressure in the lungs is greater in the lungs than the atmosphere. At rest the normal exhalation is a passive process as no skeletal muscle are involved in the process. The process results from elastic recoil of the chest walls and the lungs (Figure 23.2).

Exhalation increases during certain activities such as exercise. During exercise, the muscles of exhalation, which are the abdominals and intercostal muscles, contract thus increasing the abdominal and the thoracic region.

As the abdominal muscle contracts, the inferior ribs move downwards and compress the abdominal viscera, and the diaphragm moves upwards (Figure 23.2).

Factors affecting pulmonary ventilation
Surface tension of alveolar fluid

Surface tension is provided by the fluid called surfactant, which is a mixture of phospholipids and lipoproteins. During inhalation the surface tension must be overcome to expand the lungs and it also aids in the lungs' elastic recoil.

Airway resistance

The flow of air through the airway passage depends on the resistance and pressure difference. The walls of the airways offer some resistance to the flow of air into and out of the lungs. During inspirations the bronchioles dilate because their walls are pulled in all directions. The diameter of the airway passage is also dependent on the smooth muscles. Stimulation from the sympathetic nerve fibres causes the smooth muscles to relax resulting in bronchodilation and decreased resistance.

Compliance of the lungs

Compliance means the effort that is needed for lung and chest expansion. The higher the compliance the less effort is needed in chest and lung expansion, and low compliance means that more effort is needed. In the lungs there are two factors that play a part in compliance: the surface tension and elasticity.

Normal lungs have a high compliance and expand easily because the elastic fibres stretch readily and surfactant in the lungs reduces surface tension. In pulmonary diseases, for example emphysema, there is decreased compliance due to loss of elastic fibres of the alveolar walls.

Lung volumes

A healthy adult at rest normally has a respiration rate of 12–18 breaths per minute and with each respiration 500 ml of air is moved in or out of the lungs. The volume of air in one breath is called tidal volume. By taking a deep breath, you can increase the tidal volume above 500 ml (inspiratory reserve volume). In adult males this could be up to 3100 ml and in females it is approximately 1900 ml.

24 Control of breathing

Figure 24.1 Respiratory centre

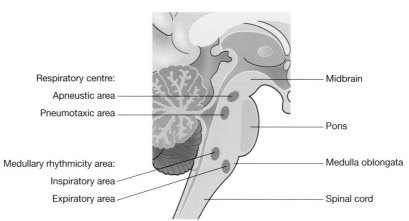

Respiratory centre:
Apneustic area
Pneumotaxic area

Medullary rhythmicity area:
Inspiratory area
Expiratory area

Midbrain
Pons
Medulla oblongata
Spinal cord

Source: Peate I, Wild K & Nair M (eds) Nursing Practice: Knowledge and Care (2014)

Figure 24.2 Peripheral chemoreceptors

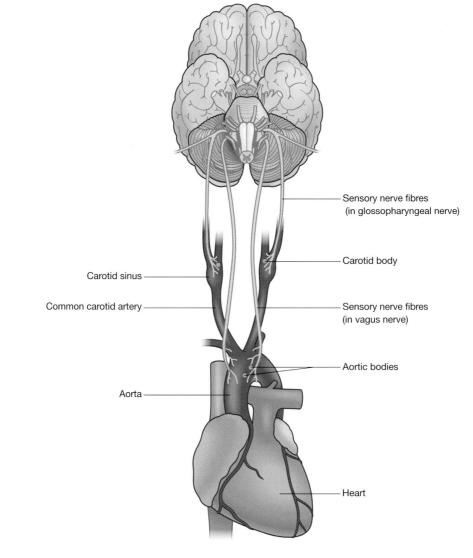

Sensory nerve fibres
(in glossopharyngeal nerve)

Carotid body

Carotid sinus

Common carotid artery

Sensory nerve fibres
(in vagus nerve)

Aortic bodies

Aorta

Heart

Pneumotaxic area

Another important area of the respiratory centre is the pneumotaxic area (Figure 24.1). This area is in the pons and is important for regulating the amount of air one takes in with each breath. Yet, the inspiratory musculature is controlled by the dorsal respiratory group. So, this is where the pneumotaxic area comes into play. The pneumotaxic area alters the bursting pattern of the dorsal respiratory group. When we find ourselves needing to breathe faster, the pneumotaxic area tells the dorsal respiratory group to speed it up. And when we need to take longer breaths, the pneumotaxic area tells the dorsal respiratory group to prolong its bursts. All the information from the body that needs to feed into the control of our breathing converges in the pneumotaxic area, so that it can properly adjust our breathing.

Apneustic area

Another part of the brain that coordinates transition between inhalation and exhalation is the apneustic area. This is situated in the lower pons (Figure 24.1). This area sends signals to the inspiratory area that activate and prolong inhalation, resulting in long, deep inhalation. When the pneumotaxic area is active, it overrides the signals from the apneustic area.

Medullary rhythmicity area

The function of this area is to control the respiratory rhythm. There are inspiratory and expiratory areas within the medullary rhythmicity area (Figure 23.1). During quiet breathing, the inhalation is about 2 seconds while the expiration is 3 seconds. Impulses from the inspiratory area maintain this rhythm. When the inspiratory area is active, the expiratory area is inactive.

However, during forceful breathing the expiratory area is stimulated by nerves from inspiratory area. Stimulation by the expiratory area causes the intercostal and abdominal to contract, which causes a decrease in the thoracic cavity and forceful exhalation.

Central chemoreceptors

These areas are found in the brain stem, and contain neurons within them, central chemoreceptors, that detect changes in the carbon dioxide levels. The way they do this is somewhat indirect. When the carbon dioxide levels rise, that means that the respiration rate has to increase, getting rid of the carbon dioxide and taking in more oxygen. Carbon dioxide does not tend to remain CO_2 gas in water. Instead, it changes into a bicarbonate ion, producing hydrogen ions as a by-product of this conversion.

In blood, when carbon dioxide is converted into bicarbonate ions, the hydrogen ions are not a problem because they immediately associate with haemoglobin (the globin act to buffer the hydrogen ions). However, in the brain, in the chemosensitive areas, there is no haemoglobin. The cerebrospinal fluid of the brain does not have proteins to buffer the hydrogen ions. So when levels of CO_2 in the brain begin to increase, much of it is converted into bicarbonate ions and hydrogen ions. The central chemoreceptors are sensitive to hydrogen ion levels. So they indirectly recognise the increase in carbon dioxide levels.

However, a change in plasma pH alone will not stimulate central chemoreceptors as H+ are not be able to diffuse across the blood–brain barrier into the CSF. Only CO_2 levels affect this as it can diffuse across, reacting with H_2O to form carbonic acid and thus decrease pH. Central chemoreception remains, in this way, distinct from peripheral chemoreceptors.

Peripheral chemoreceptors

These are not quite as important as the central chemoreceptors. Where the common carotid artery branches into the internal and external carotid arteries, there is a small swelling (Figure 24.2). This swelling is the carotid sinus, and it contains regions called carotid bodies within it. The aorta contains regions called aortic bodies within it. These regions contain our peripheral chemoreceptors, which detect oxygen levels directly. Exactly how these neurons can be sensitive to oxygen isn't the issue here, but instead, it is interesting to note that these neurons can only detect large decreases in oxygen levels; so they are only activated when oxygen levels drop to very low, life-threatening situations.

Each carotid body is a few millimetres in size and has the distinction of having the highest blood flow per tissue weight of any organ in the body. Afferent nerve fibres join with the sinus nerve before entering the glossopharyngeal nerve. A decrease in carotid body blood flow results in cellular hypoxia, hypercapnia and decreased pH that lead to an increase in receptor stimulation.

Inflation reflex

This reflex, like most, is a type of negative feedback. As the lungs expand, there are sensory neurons that detect lung stretching; stretch receptors, but they are not at all like the stretch receptors in muscle. These neurons are sensory neurons that detect stretch. The more these neurons are active, the more they send signals into the pneumotaxic area and tell it to end this round of inspiration. That prevents the lungs from ever overinflating.

Other influences on respiration
Limbic system

Can increase rate and depth of ventilation in times of stress through inspiratory area stimulation.

Temperature

An increase or decrease in body temperature can increase or decrease the respiration rate, for example fever and hypothermia, respectively.

Pain

A sudden severe pain can cause a brief period of apnoea while a prolonged somatic pain increases the respiration rate.

Irritation of airways

Cessation of breathing can result from physical or chemical irritation of the pharynx. This is followed by coughing and sneezing.

25 Gas exchange

Figure 25.1 External respiration

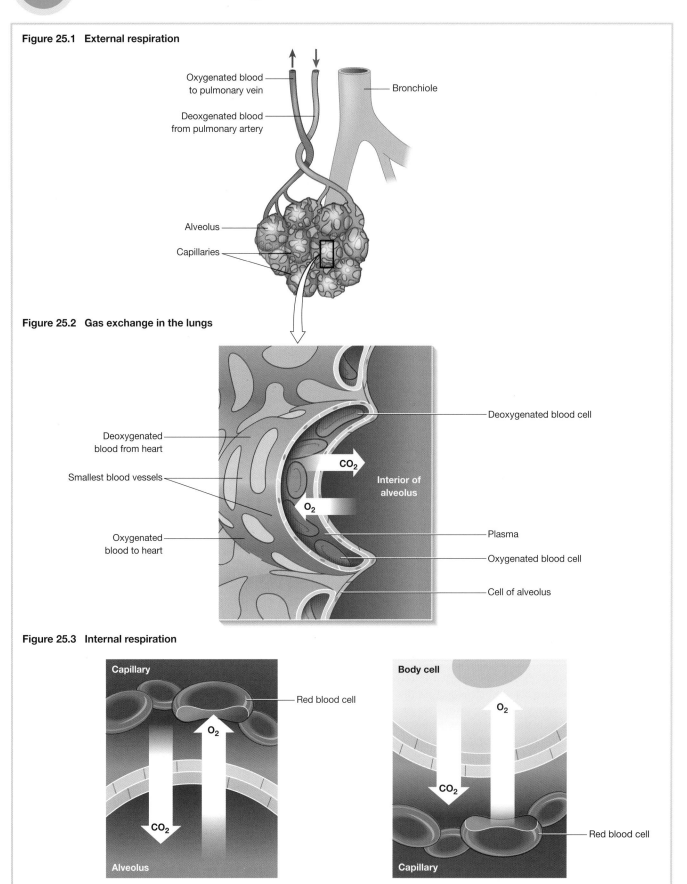

Oxygenated blood
to pulmonary vein

Deoxgenated blood
from pulmonary artery

Bronchiole

Alveolus

Capillaries

Figure 25.2 Gas exchange in the lungs

Deoxygenated
blood from heart

Smallest blood vessels

Oxygenated
blood to heart

Deoxygenated blood cell

CO_2

Interior of
alveolus

O_2

Plasma

Oxygenated blood cell

Cell of alveolus

Figure 25.3 Internal respiration

Capillary

Red blood cell

O_2

CO_2

Alveolus

Body cell

O_2

CO_2

Red blood cell

Capillary

Anatomy and Physiology for Nurses at a Glance, First Edition. Ian Peate and Muralitharan Nair. © 2015 John Wiley & Sons, Ltd. Published 2015 by John Wiley & Sons, Ltd.
Companion website: www.ataglanceseries.com/nursing/anatomy

External respiration

External respiration (pulmonary gas exchange) is the diffusion of oxygen from the alveolar sac to the lung capillaries and the diffusion of carbon dioxide from the lung capillaries to the alveolar sac to be exhaled. External respiration converts the oxygenated blood in the lungs to oxygenated blood before the blood returns to the left side of the heart.

External respiration only occurs beyond the respiratory bronchioles. For this reason the end portion of the bronchial tree is called the respiratory zone. The remainder of the bronchial tree from the trachea down to the terminal bronchioles is the conducting zone. External respiration is the diffusion of oxygen from the alveoli into pulmonary circulation (blood flow through the lungs) and the diffusion of carbon dioxide in the opposite direction (Figure 25.1). Diffusion occurs because gas molecules always move from areas of high concentration to low concentration.

Exchange of gases in the lungs

Exchange of gases in the lungs takes place between alveolar air and the blood flowing through the lung capillaries (Figure 25.2). Before oxygen can enter the internal environment and before carbon dioxide can leave the internal environment they must cross the capillary and alveolar membranes. Oxygen enters the blood from the alveolar sac because the PO_2 of alveolar air is greater than the PO_2 of incoming blood. Simultaneously, carbon dioxide molecules leave the blood by diffusing down the carbon dioxide pressure gradient out into the alveolar sac. The PCO_2 of venous blood is much higher than the PCO_2 of alveolar air.

Fick's Law

Fick's Law is a principle that describes the movement of gases (oxygen and carbon dioxide) across the respiratory membrane of the alveoli. This is explained by the following formula:

$$J = (S/wt_{mol}) \times A \times \Delta C/t$$

J = Rate of diffusion
S/wt_{mol} = Solubility/molecular weight
A = Surface area
ΔC = Concentration difference
t = Membrane thickness

It takes approximately 0.25 seconds for an oxygen molecule to diffuse from the alveoli into pulmonary circulation. However there are various influencing factors that determine the rate by which oxygen and carbon dioxide diffuse between alveoli and pulmonary circulation. Thus it could be said that the diffusion of gases is more efficient if the surface area is large, if the thickness of the membrane is small, the solubility of gas if high and the partial pressure gradient is high.

Internal respiration

Internal respiration describes the exchange of oxygen and carbon dioxide between blood and tissue cells (Figure 25.3); a phenomenon governed by the same principles as external respiration. Cells utilise oxygen when manufacturing the cells' prime energy source, adenosine tri-phosphate (ATP). In addition to ATP the cells also produce water and carbon dioxide. Because cells are continually using oxygen, its concentration within tissues is always lower than within blood. Likewise the continual use of oxygen ensures that the level of carbon dioxide within a tissue is always higher than within blood. As blood flows through the capillaries, oxygen and carbon dioxide follow their pressure gradients and continually diffuse between blood and tissue. The concentration of oxygen in blood flowing away from the tissues, back towards the heart is described as being deoxygenated. In reality if measured, the oxygen saturation of venous blood would probably be around 75%. This means that only around 25% of oxygen content (CaO_2) leaves the bloodstream, leaving a plentiful supply.

Factors affecting pulmonary and systemic gas exchange

Partial pressure difference of gases

Alveolar PO_2 has got to be greater than the blood PO_2 for oxygen to diffuse out from the alveolar sac into the lung capillaries. Certain factors, such as exercise and drugs, can affect the rate of diffusion. Morphine slows the rate of ventilation thus affecting gas exchange in the lungs.

Surface area available for gas exchange

A pulmonary disorder can affect gas exchange. Conditions such as emphysema and carcinoma of the lungs can result in poor ventilation. In emphysema, alveolar walls are destroyed and there are few functional alveolar sacs available for gas exchange.

Diffusion distance

Normally, gas exchange within the lungs occurs without any problem as the alveolar and lung capillaries are in close proximity. Gases move in and out readily; however, when the person suffers from conditions such pulmonary oedema, the gas exchange is affected. Fluid fills in the alveolar sac making the distance greater and thus slowing down the gas exchange.

Solubility of gases

Oxygen has a lower molecular weight compared to carbon dioxide and thus diffuses at a greater rate. However, carbon dioxide is much more soluble in fluid then oxygen, thus the net movement of carbon dioxide is far greater than the net inward movement of oxygen.

Transport of gases

Both oxygen (O_2) and carbon dioxide are transported from the lungs to the body tissues in blood. Both gases travel in blood plasma and haemoglobin, which is found within erythrocytes (red blood cells). Each erythrocyte contains approximately 280 million haemoglobin molecules and each haemoglobin has the potential to carry four O_2 molecules. The delivery of oxygen, therefore, is also reliant upon the presence of an adequate supply of erythrocytes and haemoglobin (Hb).

Just like oxygen, a small amount of carbon dioxide (CO_2), around 10%, is transported in plasma. Carbon dioxide is also transported attached to haemoglobin (Hb), although only around 30% is transported that way.

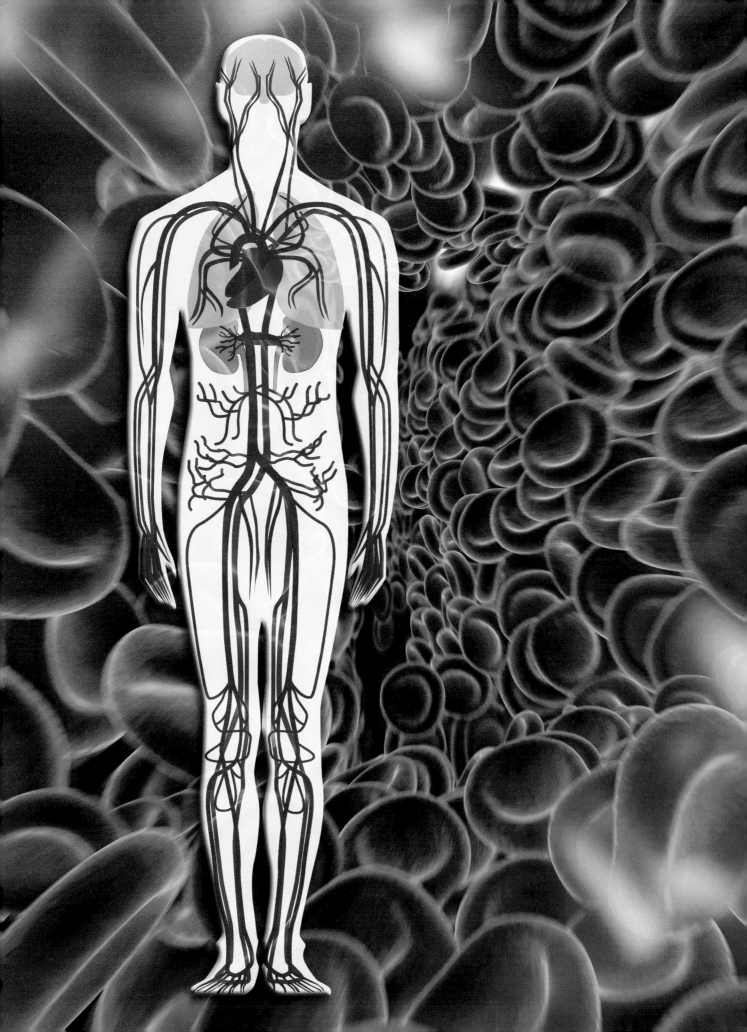

The gastrointestinal tract

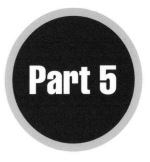

Part 5

Chapters

26 The upper gastrointestinal tract

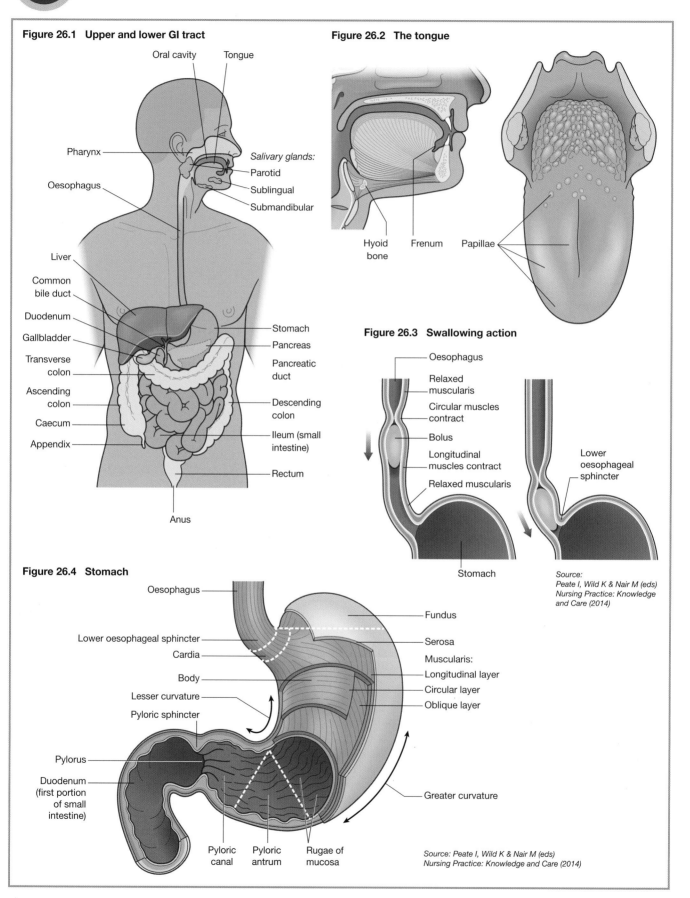

Figure 26.1 Upper and lower GI tract

- Oral cavity
- Tongue
- Pharynx
- Oesophagus
- Salivary glands:
  - Parotid
  - Sublingual
  - Submandibular
- Liver
- Common bile duct
- Duodenum
- Gallbladder
- Transverse colon
- Ascending colon
- Caecum
- Appendix
- Stomach
- Pancreas
- Pancreatic duct
- Descending colon
- Ileum (small intestine)
- Rectum
- Anus

Figure 26.2 The tongue

- Hyoid bone
- Frenum
- Papillae

Figure 26.3 Swallowing action

- Oesophagus
- Relaxed muscularis
- Circular muscles contract
- Bolus
- Longitudinal muscles contract
- Relaxed muscularis
- Lower oesophageal sphincter
- Stomach

Source:
Peate I, Wild K & Nair M (eds)
Nursing Practice: Knowledge
and Care (2014)

Figure 26.4 Stomach

- Oesophagus
- Lower oesophageal sphincter
- Cardia
- Body
- Lesser curvature
- Pyloric sphincter
- Pylorus
- Duodenum (first portion of small intestine)
- Pyloric canal
- Pyloric antrum
- Rugae of mucosa
- Fundus
- Serosa
- Muscularis:
  - Longitudinal layer
  - Circular layer
  - Oblique layer
- Greater curvature

Source: Peate I, Wild K & Nair M (eds)
Nursing Practice: Knowledge and Care (2014)

Anatomy and Physiology for Nurses at a Glance, First Edition. Ian Peate and Muralitharan Nair. © 2015 John Wiley & Sons, Ltd. Published 2015 by John Wiley & Sons, Ltd.
Companion website: www.ataglanceseries.com/nursing/anatomy

The mouth (oral cavity)

The mouth or oral cavity is where the process of digestion begins (Figure 26.1). The oral cavity consists of several different structures. The lips and cheeks are muscular and connective tissue structures, lined with mucus-secreting, stratified squamous epithelial cells which provide protection against abrasion caused by wear and tear.

Lips and cheeks

The lips and cheeks help to move and hold food in the mouth while the teeth tear and grind the food. This process is called mastication (chewing). The lips and cheeks are also involved in speech and facial expression.

Tongue

The tongue is a muscular organ in the mouth. The tongue is covered with moist, pink tissue called mucosa. Tiny bumps called papillae give the tongue its rough texture. Thousands of taste buds cover the surfaces of the papillae. Taste buds are collections of nerve-like cells that connect to nerves running into the brain. The tongue is anchored to the mouth by webs of tough tissue and mucosa. The tether holding down the front of the tongue is called the frenum (Figure 26.2). In the back of the mouth, the tongue is anchored into the hyoid bone. The tongue is vital for chewing and swallowing food, as well as for speech.

Palate

The palate forms the roof of the mouth and consists of two parts: the hard palate and the soft palate. The hard palate is located anteriorly and is bony. The soft palate lies posteriorly and consists of skeletal muscle and connective tissue. The palate plays a part in swallowing. The palatine tonsils lie laterally and are lymphoid tissue. The uvula is a fold of tissue that hangs down from the centre of the soft palate.

Salivary glands

Saliva is produced in and secreted from salivary glands. The basic secretory units of salivary glands are clusters of cells called acini. These cells secrete a fluid that contains water, electrolytes, mucus and enzymes, all of which flow out of the acinus into collecting ducts.

Within the ducts, the composition of the secretion is altered. Much of the sodium is actively reabsorbed, potassium is secreted, and large quantities of bicarbonate ion are secreted. Bicarbonate is important because it, along with phosphate, provides a critical buffer that neutralizes the massive quantities of acid produced in the stomach.

Oesophagus

When food exits the oropharynx it enters the oesophagus. The oesophagus extends from the laryngopharynx to the stomach. It is a thick walled structure and measures about 25 cm in length and lies in the thoracic cavity, posterior to the trachea. The function of the oesophagus is to transport substances (the food bolus) from the mouth to the stomach. Thick mucous is secreted by the mucosa of the oesophagus and this aids the passage of the food bolus and protects the oesophagus from abrasion.

The upper oesophageal sphincter regulates the movement of substances into the oesophagus and the lower oesophageal sphincter (also known as the cardiac sphincter) regulates the movement of substances from the oesophagus to the stomach. The muscle layer of the oesophagus differs from the rest of the digestive tract as the superior portion consists of skeletal (voluntary) muscle and the inferior portion consists of smooth (involuntary) muscle. Breathing and swallowing cannot occur at the same time.

Swallowing (deglutition)

Swallowing occurs in three phases: the voluntary phase is where food is moved to the oropharynx by the voluntary muscle. Next is the pharyngeal phase which is under the involuntary neuromuscular control. Once the food bolus encroaches on the palatoglossal folds, or anterior tonsilar pillars, the pharyngeal phase of swallowing reflexively begins.

The third phase is the oesophageal phase. Like the pharyngeal phase of swallowing, the oesophageal phase of swallowing is under involuntary neuromuscular control. The outer fibres of the upper zone are arranged longitudinally while the inner fibres have a circular configuration (Figure 26.3).

Stomach

The stomach is a muscular organ located on the left side of the upper abdomen. The stomach receives food from the oesophagus. As food reaches the end of the oesophagus, it enters the stomach through a muscular valve called the lower oesophageal sphincter (Figure 26.4).

The stomach is supplied with arterial blood from a branch of the celiac artery and venous blood leaves the stomach via the hepatic vein. The vagus nerve innervates the stomach with parasympathetic fibres that stimulate gastric motility and the secretion of gastric juice. Sympathetic fibres from the celiac plexus reduce gastric activity.

The stomach has the same four layers of tissue as the digestive tract but with some differences. The muscularis contains three layers of smooth muscle instead of two. It has longitudinal, circular and oblique muscle fibres. The extra muscle layer facilitates the churning, mixing and mechanical breakdown of food that occurs within the stomach as well as supporting the onward journey of the food by peristalsis.

The stomach secretes acid and enzymes that digest food. Ridges of muscle tissue called rugae line the stomach. The stomach muscles contract periodically, churning food to enhance digestion. The pyloric sphincter is a muscular valve that opens to allow food to pass from the stomach to the duodenum.

27 The lower gastrointestinal tract

Figure 27.1 Small intestine

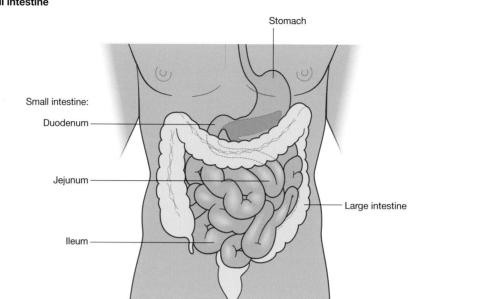

Stomach

Small intestine:

Duodenum

Jejunum

Large intestine

Ileum

Source: Peate I, Wild K & Nair M (eds) Nursing Practice: Knowledge and Care (2014)

Figure 27.2 Large intestine

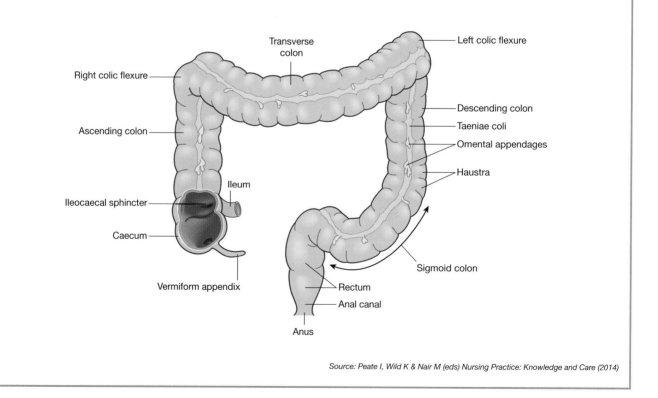

Transverse colon

Left colic flexure

Right colic flexure

Descending colon

Taeniae coli

Omental appendages

Ascending colon

Haustra

Ileum

Ileocaecal sphincter

Caecum

Vermiform appendix

Sigmoid colon

Rectum

Anal canal

Anus

Source: Peate I, Wild K & Nair M (eds) Nursing Practice: Knowledge and Care (2014)

Anatomy and Physiology for Nurses at a Glance, First Edition. Ian Peate and Muralitharan Nair. © 2015 John Wiley & Sons, Ltd. Published 2015 by John Wiley & Sons, Ltd.
Companion website: www.ataglanceseries.com/nursing/anatomy

Small intestine

The small intestine is the part of the gastrointestinal tract following the stomach, and is where much of the digestion and absorption of food takes place. The small intestine consists of three sections. The first portion, called the duodenum, connects to the stomach. The middle portion is the jejunum. The final section, called the ileum, attaches to the large intestine (Figure 27.1).

The small intestine is innervated with both parasympathetic (from the vagus nerve) and parasympathetic (from the thoracic splanchnic nerve) systems. It receives its arterial blood supply from the superior mesenteric artery and nutrient-rich venous blood drains into the superior mesenteric vein and eventually into the hepatic portal vein toward the liver.

Duodenum

The duodenum is a short portion of the small intestine connecting it to the stomach (Figure 27.1). It is approximately 25 cm long, while the entire small intestine measures about 6.5 metres. This structure begins with the duodenal bulb, bordered by the pyloric sphincter that marks the lower end of the stomach, and is connected by the ligament of Treitz to the diaphragm before leading into the next portion of the small intestine, the jejunum.

The duodenum is largely responsible for the breakdown of food in the small intestine, using enzymes. The villi of the duodenum have a leafy-looking appearance, a histologically identifiable structure. Brunner's glands, which secrete mucus, are found in the duodenum. The duodenum wall is composed of a very thin layer of cells that form the muscularis mucosae.

The duodenum also regulates the rate of emptying of the stomach. Secretin and cholecystokinin are released from cells in the duodenal epithelium in response to acidic and fatty stimuli present there when the pylorus opens and releases gastric chyme into the duodenum for further digestion. These cause the liver and gall bladder to release bile, and the pancreas to release bicarbonate and digestive enzymes such as trypsin, lipase and amylase into the duodenum as they are needed.

Jejunum

The section of the small intestine that comprises the first two-fifths beyond the duodenum; it is larger, thicker-walled, and more vascular and has more circular folds than the ileum.

The inner surface of the jejunum, its mucous membrane, is covered in projections called villi, which increase the surface area of tissue available to absorb nutrients from the gut contents. The epithelial cells which line these villi possess even larger numbers of microvilli. The transport of nutrients across epithelial cells through the jejunum and ileum includes the passive transport of sugar fructose and the active transport of amino acids, small peptides, vitamins and most glucose. The villi in the jejunum are much longer than in the duodenum or ileum.

The jejunum contains very few Brunner's glands (found in the duodenum) or Peyer's patches (found in the ileum). However, there are a few jejunal lymph nodes suspended in its mesentery. The jejunum has many large circular folds in its submucosa called plicae circulares, which increase the surface area for nutrient absorption.

Ileum

The ileum is the final and longest segment of the small intestine. It is specifically responsible for the absorption of vitamin B_{12} and the reabsorption of conjugated bile salts. The ileum is about 4 metres long and extends from the jejunum (the middle section of the small intestine) to the ileocecal valve, which empties into the colon (large intestine). The ileum is suspended from the abdominal wall by the mesentery, a fold of serous membrane.

The smooth muscle of the ileum is thinner than the walls of other parts of the intestine, and its peristaltic contractions are slower. The ileum's lining is also less permeable than that of the upper small intestine. Small collections of lymphatic tissue (Peyer patches) are embedded in the ileal wall, and specific receptors for bile salts and vitamin B_{12} are contained exclusively in its lining; about 90% of the conjugated bile salts in the intestinal contents is absorbed by the ileum.

Large intestine (colon)

The large intestine, the posterior section of the intestine, consists of four regions: the cecum, colon, rectum and anus (Figure 27.2). The term colon is sometimes used to refer to the entire large intestine. The large intestine is wider and shorter than the small intestine (approximately 1.5 metres in length) and has a smooth inner wall. In the upper half of the large intestine, enzymes from the small intestine complete the digestive process, and bacteria produce B vitamins (B_{12}, thiamin and riboflavin).

The large intestine mucosa contains large numbers of goblet cells that secrete mucus to ease the passage of faeces and protect the walls of the colon. The simple columnar epithelium changes to stratified squamous epithelium at the anal canal. Anal sinuses secrete mucus in response to faecal compression. This protects the anal canal from the abrasion associated with emptying.

The food residue from the ileum is fluid when in enters the caecum and contains very few nutrients. The small intestine is responsible for some of the absorption of water but the primary function of the large intestine is to absorb water and turn the food residue into semi solid faeces. The large intestine also absorbs some vitamins, minerals, electrolytes and drugs.

28 The liver, gallbladder and biliary tree

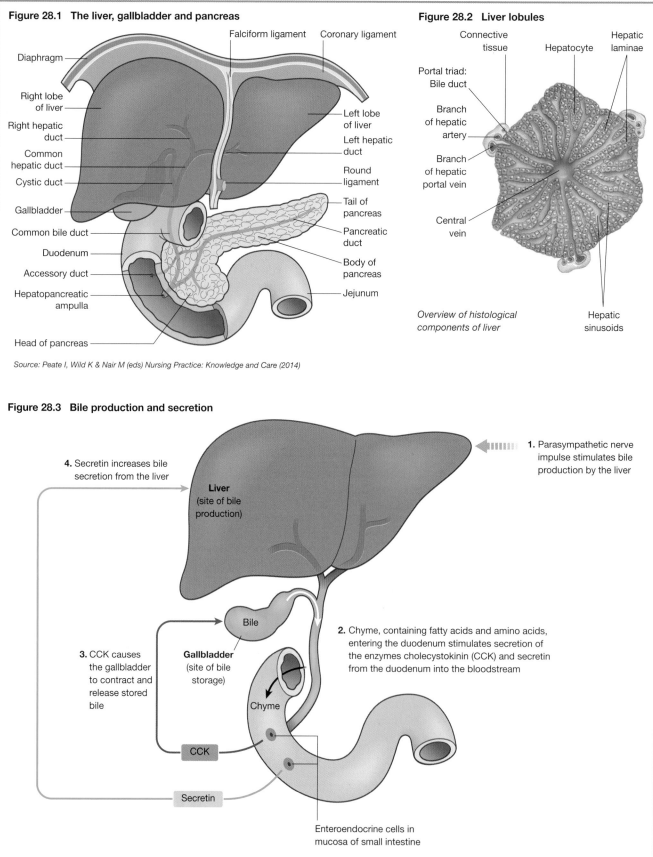

Figure 28.1 The liver, gallbladder and pancreas

- Diaphragm
- Falciform ligament
- Coronary ligament
- Right lobe of liver
- Right hepatic duct
- Common hepatic duct
- Cystic duct
- Gallbladder
- Common bile duct
- Duodenum
- Accessory duct
- Hepatopancreatic ampulla
- Head of pancreas
- Left lobe of liver
- Left hepatic duct
- Round ligament
- Tail of pancreas
- Pancreatic duct
- Body of pancreas
- Jejunum

Source: Peate I, Wild K & Nair M (eds) Nursing Practice: Knowledge and Care (2014)

Figure 28.2 Liver lobules

- Connective tissue
- Hepatocyte
- Hepatic laminae
- Portal triad:
  - Bile duct
  - Branch of hepatic artery
  - Branch of hepatic portal vein
- Central vein
- Hepatic sinusoids

Overview of histological components of liver

Figure 28.3 Bile production and secretion

4. Secretin increases bile secretion from the liver

Liver (site of bile production)

1. Parasympathetic nerve impulse stimulates bile production by the liver

3. CCK causes the gallbladder to contract and release stored bile

Bile

Gallbladder (site of bile storage)

Chyme

2. Chyme, containing fatty acids and amino acids, entering the duodenum stimulates secretion of the enzymes cholecystokinin (CCK) and secretin from the duodenum into the bloodstream

CCK

Secretin

Enteroendocrine cells in mucosa of small intestine

Anatomy and Physiology for Nurses at a Glance, First Edition. Ian Peate and Muralitharan Nair. © 2015 John Wiley & Sons, Ltd. Published 2015 by John Wiley & Sons, Ltd.
Companion website: www.ataglanceseries.com/nursing/anatomy

Liver

The liver is the largest solid organ in the body. In adults, the liver can weigh up to 1.5 kilograms (kg). It is in the upper-right abdomen, just under the rib cage and below the diaphragm (the thin muscle below the lungs and heart that separates the chest cavity from the abdomen.

Two major types of cells populate the liver lobes: karat parenchymal and non-parenchymal cells: 80% of the liver volume is occupied by parenchymal cells commonly referred to as hepatocytes. Non-parenchymal cells constitute 40% of the total number of liver cells but only 6.5% of its volume.

Segments of the liver

The liver is divided into segments (Figure 28.1). Each segment of the liver is further divided into lobules. Lobules are usually represented as discrete hexagonal aggregations of hepatocytes. The hepatocytes assemble as plates which radiate from a central vein. Lobules are served by arterial, venous and biliary vessels at their periphery. Human lung lobules have little connective tissue separating one lobule from another. The paucity of connective tissue makes it more difficult to identify the portal triads and the boundaries of individual lobules. Central veins are easier to identify due to their large lumen and because they lack connective tissue that invests the portal triad vessels.

Ligaments of the liver

The coronary ligament attaches the liver (from the diaphragmatic surface) to the diaphragm. It is an irregular fold of peritoneum. It surrounds the triangular base of the diaphragmatic surface. It is continuous with outer most layer of the caudal vena cava. The falciform ligament is ventral to the coronary ligament. It is located cranial to the umbilicus and is a vestige of the umbilical vein. The triangular ligament is on the right and left sides of the coronary ligament.

Blood supply

The liver gets a dual blood supply both from the hepatic portal vein and hepatic arteries. The hepatic portal vein supplies 75% of the blood supply. This venous blood is drained from the spleen, gastrointestinal tract and other organs. The hepatic arteries supply arterial blood to the liver, accounting for the remainder of its blood flow. Oxygen is provided from both vessels; approximately half of the liver's oxygen demand is met by the hepatic portal vein and half by the hepatic arteries.

The hepatic artery comes off the celiac trunk which in turn comes from the aorta. The venous blood from the digestive tract is collected by the portal vein, which then supplies blood to liver. The hepatic veins drain blood from liver into the inferior vena cava. Branches of the hepatic artery and vein and the bile duct flow into the liver. Collectively, these three vessels are termed the portal triad and they are located at the corners of the liver lobules (Figure 28.2).

Liver functions

Nearly all the blood circulated around the abdomen flows back through the portal vein to the liver where it comes in contact with the liver cells, ensuring the products of digestion are presented to the hepatic cells before entering the general circulation. Other functions include production of bile, carbohydrate metabolism, glycogenesis, glyconeolysis, gluconeogenesis and the breakdown of insulin and other hormones. Protein metabolism produces soluble mediators of the clotting cascade, albumin and hormone transporting globulins. The liver is also involved in lipid metabolism, lipogenesis and the synthesis of cholesterol.

It also has a role in immunoregulation via Kupfer cells and the complement synthesis and metabolism. The liver is important in storage of water-soluble vitamins, fat-soluble vitamins, iron, triglyceride and glycogen.

The liver breaks down haemoglobin and toxic substances through drug metabolism. It converts ammonia to urea and regulates the management of wastes of metabolism, such as haem and ammonia (amino acids).

Gallbladder

The gallbladder is a small green muscular sac that lies posterior to the liver (Figure 28.2). It functions as a reservoir for bile until it is needed for digestion. It also concentrates bile by absorbing water. The mucosa of the gallbladder, like the rugae of the stomach, contain folds that allow the gallbladder to stretch in order to accommodate varying volumes of bile. When the smooth muscle walls of the gallbladder contract, bile is expelled into the cystic duct and down into the common bile duct before entering the duodenum via the hepatopancreatic ampulla.

Function of bile

When food containing fat enters the digestive tract, it stimulates the secretion of cholecystokinin (CCK). In response to CCK, the adult human gallbladder, which stores approximately 50 millilitres of bile, releases the bile into the duodenum. The bile emulsifies fats in partly digested food. During storage in the gallbladder, bile becomes more concentrated which increases its potency and intensifies its effect on fats (Figure 28.3).

Biliary tree (tract)

The biliary tract (or biliary tree) is the term for the path by which bile is secreted by the liver then transported to the first part of the small intestine, also known as the duodenum. It is referred to as a tree because it begins with many small branches which end in the common bile duct, sometimes referred to as the trunk of the biliary tree (Figure 28.3).

29 Pancreas and spleen

Figure 29.1 The pancreas

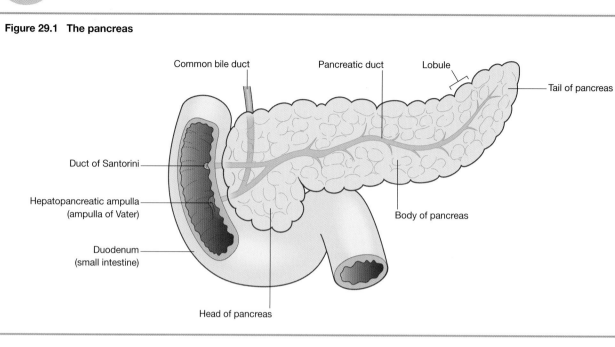

Common bile duct

Pancreatic duct

Lobule

Tail of pancreas

Duct of Santorini

Hepatopancreatic ampulla
(ampulla of Vater)

Duodenum
(small intestine)

Body of pancreas

Head of pancreas

Anatomy and Physiology for Nurses at a Glance, First Edition. Ian Peate and Muralitharan Nair. © 2015 John Wiley & Sons, Ltd. Published 2015 by John Wiley & Sons, Ltd.
Companion website: www.ataglanceseries.com/nursing/anatomy

Pancreas

The pancreas is approximately 12–15 cm long and 2.5 cm thick. It is situated across the back of the abdomen, behind the stomach. The head of the pancreas is on the right side of the abdomen and it is connected to the duodenum (the first section of the small intestine) through a small tube called the pancreatic duct. The narrow end of the pancreas, called the tail, extends to the left side of the body (Figure 29.1).

The pancreatic juices are secreted by exocrine cells into small ducts that unite to form larger ducts. The duct of Wirsung is the larger of the two ducts and in most people this duct joins the common bile duct and enters the duodenum as a dilated common duct called the hepatopancreatic ampulla. In most people there is a second smaller (minor or accessory) papilla, situated about 2 cm above the main papilla, and slightly to its right. This is the exit place for Santorini's duct. The minor papilla occasionally takes over when the main papilla is not able to function correctly and becomes the main site of drainage for pancreatic juices.

The cells of the pancreas are responsible for making the endocrine and exocrine products. The islet cells of the islets of Langerhans produce the endocrine hormones insulin and glucagon. These hormones control carbohydrate metabolism.

Composition of pancreatic juice

Two hormones regulate the secretion of pancreatic juice. Secretin, produced in response to the presence of hydrochloric acid in the duodenum, promotes the secretion of bicarbonate ions. Cholecystokinin, secreted in response to the intake of protein and fat, promotes the secretion of the enzymes present in pancreatic juice. Parasympathetic vagus nerve stimulation also promotes the release of pancreatic juice.

The acini glands of the exocrine pancreas produce 1.2–1.5 l of pancreatic juice daily. Pancreatic juice is a clear colourless fluid consisting of water, mineral salts, the enzymes amylase and lipase and the inactive enzyme precursors trypsinogen, chymotrypsinogen and procarboxypeptidase. Pancreatic juice travels from the pancreas via the pancreatic duct into the duodenum at the hepatopancreatic ampulla.

The cells of the pancreatic ducts secrete bicarbonate ions which make pancreatic juice slightly alkaline pH (pH 7.1–8.2). This helps to neutralise acidic chyme from the stomach, thus protecting the small intestine from damage by the acidity, and stops the action of pepsin from the stomach. This provides a proper pH environment for the action of enzymes in the small intestine.

Functions of pancreatic juice

Functions include digestion of proteins: enteropeptidase converts trypsinogen and chymotrypsinogen into the active proteolytic enzymes trypsin and chymotrypsin. These activated enzymes convert polypeptides to tripeptides, dipeptides and amino acids. It also plays a role in digestion of carbohydrates: pancreatic amylase helps in the conversion of digestible polysaccharides (starch) not acted upon by salivary amylase to disaccharides. Bile salts help lipase in conversion of fats to fatty acids and glycerol. They do so by decreasing the size of the globules resulting in increased surface area.

Spleen

The spleen is an organ shaped like a shoe that lies relative to the 9th and 11th ribs and is located in the left hypochondrium and partly in the epigastrium. Thus, the spleen is situated between the fundus of the stomach and the diaphragm. The spleen is very vascular and reddish purple in colour; its size and weight vary.

The spleen contains two main types of tissue – white pulp and red pulp. White pulp is lymphatic tissue (material which is part of the immune system) mainly made up of white blood cells. Red pulp is made up of venous sinuses (blood-filled cavities) and splenic cords. Splenic cords are special tissues which contain different types of red and white blood cells.

The spleen has two coats; an external serous and an internal fibroelastic coat. The external or serous coat (tunica serosa) is derived from the peritoneum; it is thin, smooth, and in the human subject intimately adherent to the fibroelastic coat. It invests the entire organ, except at the hilum and along the lines of reflection of the phrenicolienal and gastrolienal ligaments.

Function of the spleen

Blood flows into the spleen where it enters the white pulp. Here, white blood cells called B and T cells screen the blood flowing through. T cells help to recognise invading pathogens (for example, bacteria and viruses) that might cause illness and then attack them. B-cells make antibodies that help to stop infections from occurring.

Blood also enters red pulp. Red pulp has three main functions. (i) It removes old and damaged red blood cells. Red blood cells have a lifespan of about 120 days. After this time they stop carrying oxygen effectively. Special cells called macrophages break down these old red blood cells. Haemoglobin (carries oxygen) found within the cells is also broken down and then recycled. (ii) Red pulp also stores up to one third of the body's supply of platelets. Platelets are fragments of cells circulating in the bloodstream that help to stop bleeding when the blood vessel is cut. These extra stored platelets can be released from the spleen if severe bleeding occurs. (iii) In foetuses red pulp can also aid in the production of new red blood cells.

The spleen is not essential to life. Other organs such as the liver and bone marrow are able to take over many of its functions.

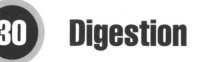

30 Digestion

Figure 30.1 Digestion and absorption

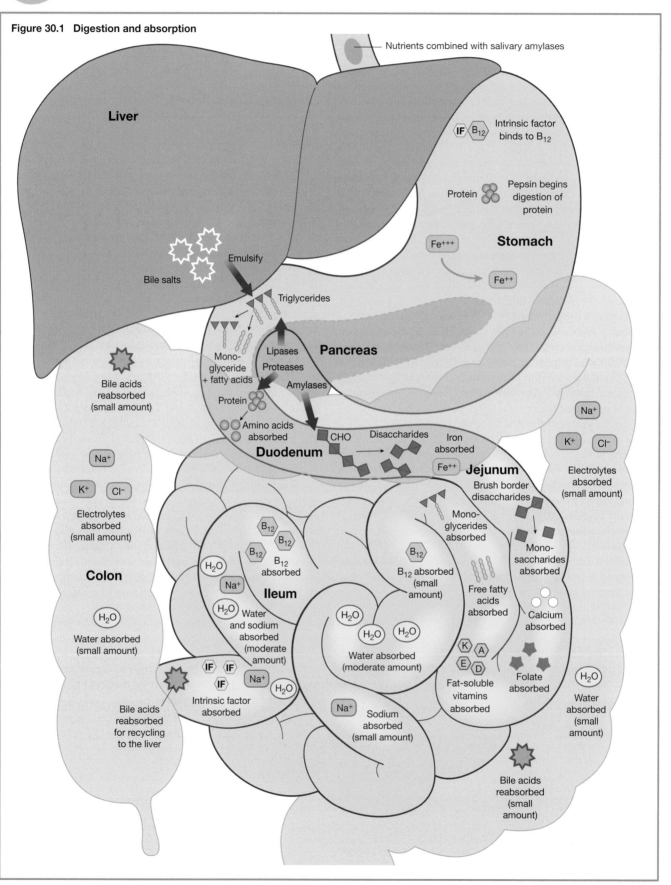

Anatomy and Physiology for Nurses at a Glance, First Edition. Ian Peate and Muralitharan Nair. © 2015 John Wiley & Sons, Ltd. Published 2015 by John Wiley & Sons, Ltd.
Companion website: www.ataglanceseries.com/nursing/anatomy

Digestion is the mechanical and chemical breaking down of food into smaller components, to a form that can be absorbed, for instance, into a blood stream. Digestion is a form of catabolism; a breakdown of macro food molecules to smaller ones (Figure 30.1).

Mechanical

Mechanical digestion is simply the aspects of digestion achieved through a mechanism or movement. There are two basic types of mechanical digestion.

Mastication

The first step when it comes to digestion actually begins as soon as food enters the mouth. Mastication (chewing) begins the process of breaking down food into nutrients. As a type of mechanical digestion, chewing our food is an important part of the digestive process because smaller pieces are more readily digested through chemical digestion.

Peristalsis

Mechanical digestion also involves the process known as peristalsis. Peristalsis is simply the involuntary contractions responsible for the movement of food through the oesophagus and intestinal tracts.

In the stomach, there are three layers of muscle. It has longitudinal, circular and oblique muscle which together contract and relax to form the churning motion which mixes food around. This aids in digestion as it slightly breaks up the food and also increases the contact the food has with enzymes and acids in the gastric juice. Bile salts also act to emulsify large fat globules into smaller fat droplets.

Chemical

Chemical digestion is achieved with the addition of chemicals to the food. Digestive enzymes and water are responsible for the breakdown of complex molecules such as fats, proteins and carbohydrates into smaller molecules. These smaller molecules can then be absorbed for use by cells.

The presence of these digestive enzymes accelerates the digestion process, where absence of these enzymes slows overall reaction speed. Digestive enzymes mainly responsible for chemical digestion include:

Protease: Any of various enzymes, including the proteinases and peptidases that catalyse the hydrolytic breakdown of proteins. Proteolytic enzymes are very important in digestion as they breakdown the peptide bonds in the protein foods to liberate the amino acids needed by the body.

Collagenase: Are enzymes that break the peptide bonds in collagen. Collagens are the major fibrous component of animal extracellular connective tissue.

Lipase: Lipids are one of the three major food groups needed for proper nutrition. Lipase is the digestive enzyme needed to digest fat. Lipase is an enzyme that hydrolyses lipids, the ester bonds in triglycerides, to form fatty acids and glycerol.

Fats require special digestive action before absorption because the end products must be carried in a water medium (blood and lymph) in which fats are not soluble. Lipase is the primary enzyme used to split fats into fatty acids and glycerol. Although little actual fat digestion occurs in the stomach, gastric lipase does digest already emulsified fats such as in egg yolk and cream.

Amylase: Any of a group of enzymes that catalyse the hydrolysis of starch to sugar to produce carbohydrate derivatives. Amylase is present in saliva, where it begins the mechanical process of digestion. Foods that contain much starch but little sugar, such as rice and potato, taste slightly sweet as they are chewed because amylase turns some of their starch into sugar in the mouth. The pancreas also makes amylase (alpha amylase) to hydrolyse dietary starch into disaccharides and trisaccharides which are converted by other enzymes to glucose to supply the body with energy.

Trypsin: A proteolytic digestive enzyme produced by the exocrine pancreas. It speeds up the chemical reaction, in the small intestine, of the breakdown of dietary proteins to peptones, peptides and amino acids. When the pancreas is stimulated by cholecystokinin, it is then secreted into the first part of the small intestine (the duodenum) via the pancreatic duct. Once in the small intestine, the enzyme enteropeptidase activates it into trypsin.

Chymotrypsin: A proteolytic enzyme produced by the pancreas that catalyses the hydrolysis of casein and gelatin. Chymotrypsin is a serine endopeptidase produced by the acinar cells of the pancreas.

Digestion and absorption

Carbohydrate: Monosaccharides, such as glucose, galactose and fructose, are produced by the breakdown of polysaccharides and are transported to the intestinal epithelium by facilitated diffusion or active transport. Facilitated diffusion moves the sugars to the bloodstream.

Protein: Proteins are broken down to peptide fragments by pepsin in the stomach, and by pancreatic trypsin and chymotrypsin in the small intestine. The fragments are then digested to free amino acids by carboxypeptidase from the pancreas and aminopeptidase from the intestinal epithelium. Free amino acids enter the epithelium by secondary active transport and leave it by facilitated diffusion. Small amounts of intact proteins can enter interstitial fluid by endo- and exocytosis.

Fat: Fat digestion occurs by pancreatic lipase in the small intestine. Large lipid droplets are first broken down into smaller droplets by a process called emulsification. Pancreatic colipase binds the water-soluble lipase to the lipid substrate.

Vitamins: Fat-soluble vitamins are absorbed and stored along with fats. Most water-soluble vitamins are absorbed by diffusion or mediated transport. Vitamin B_{12}, because of its large size and charged nature, first binds to a protein, called intrinsic factor, which is secreted by the stomach epithelium, and is then absorbed by endocytosis.

Water: Most of the material absorbed from the cavity of the small intestine is water in which salt is dissolved. The salt and water come from the food and liquid we swallow and the juices secreted by the many digestive glands.

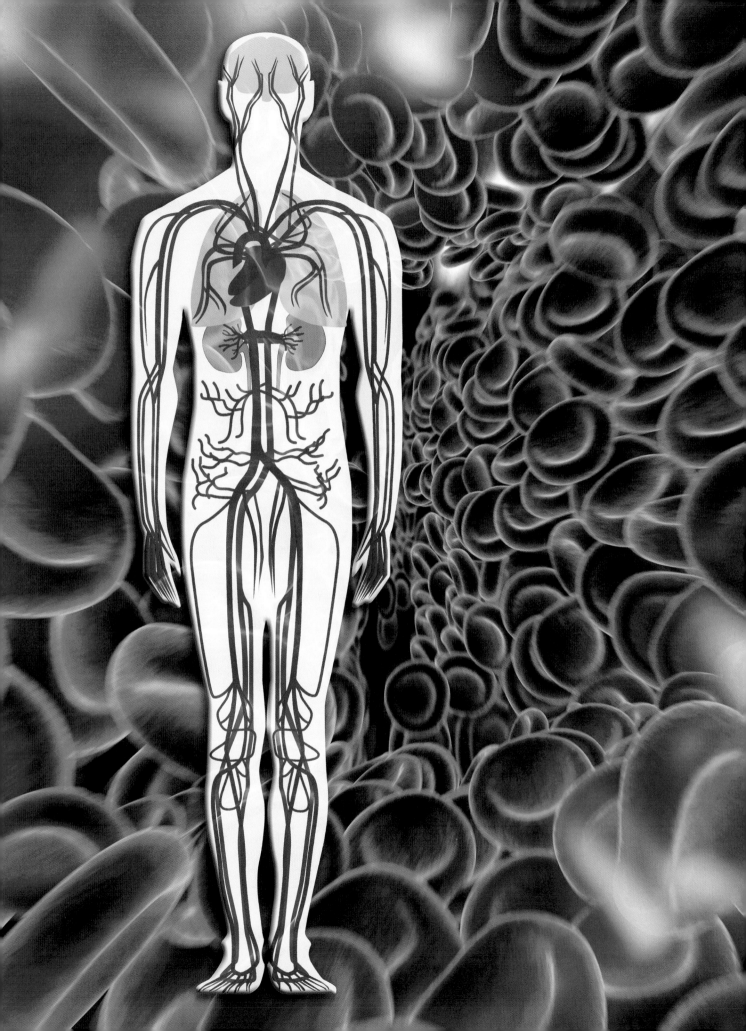

The urinary system

Part 6

Chapters

31 The kidney: microscopic

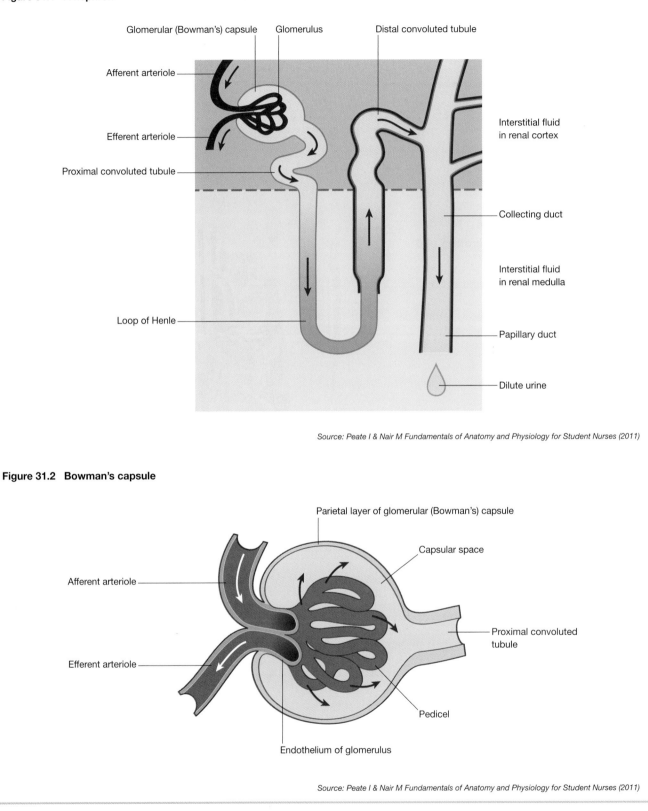

Figure 31.1 A nephron

Glomerular (Bowman's) capsule

Glomerulus

Distal convoluted tubule

Afferent arteriole

Efferent arteriole

Proximal convoluted tubule

Loop of Henle

Interstitial fluid in renal cortex

Collecting duct

Interstitial fluid in renal medulla

Papillary duct

Dilute urine

Source: Peate I & Nair M Fundamentals of Anatomy and Physiology for Student Nurses (2011)

Figure 31.2 Bowman's capsule

Parietal layer of glomerular (Bowman's) capsule

Capsular space

Afferent arteriole

Efferent arteriole

Proximal convoluted tubule

Pedicel

Endothelium of glomerulus

Source: Peate I & Nair M Fundamentals of Anatomy and Physiology for Student Nurses (2011)

Nephrons

These are small structures and they form the functional units of the kidney. The nephron consists of a glomerulus and a renal tubule (Figure 31.1). The renal tubule can be further divided into Bowman's capsule, proximal convoluted tubule, loop of Henle, distal convoluted tubule and the collecting ducts. There are approximately over one million nephrons per kidney and it is in these structures that urine is formed. Its main function is to regulate water and electrolytes by filtering the blood, reabsorbing what is needed and excreting the rest as urine. A nephron eliminates wastes from the body, regulates blood volume and blood pressure, controls levels of electrolytes and metabolites and regulates blood pH.

Glomerular capsule

Also known as glomerular capsule (Figure 31.2), this is a cup-like sac and is the first portion of the nephron. A Bowman's capsule is part of the filtration system in the kidneys. When blood reaches the kidneys for filtration, it enters the Bowman's capsule first, with the capsule separating the blood into two components: a filtrated blood product and a filtrate which is moved through the nephron, another structure in the kidneys. The glomerular capsule consists of visceral and parietal layers. The visceral layer is lined by epithelial cells called podocytes while the parietal layer is lined with simple squamous epithelium, and it is in the Bowman's capsule that the network of capillaries called the glomerulus is found.

Glomerulus

The glomerulus consists of a tight network of capillaries surrounded by podocytes. Podocytes have narrow cell processes that in turn give secondary extensions called pedicles (Figure 31.2). Podocytes completely surround the capillary network. As blood flows though the glomerulus, water and metabolic wastes are filtered through the capillary walls by the surrounding podocytes. Water and wastes pass into the Bowman's capsule.

Proximal convoluted tubule

From the Bowman's capsule, the filtrate drains into the proximal convoluted tubule (Figure 31.1). The surface of the epithelial cells of this segment of the nephron is covered with densely packed microvilli. The microvilli increase the surface area of the cells thus facilitating their resorptive function. The in-folded membranes forming the microvilli are the site of numerous sodium pumps. Reabsorption of salt, water and glucose from the glomerular filtrate occurs in this section of the tubule; at the same time certain substances, including uric acid and drug metabolites, are actively transferred from the blood capillaries into the tubule for excretion.

Loop of Henle

In the kidney, the loop of Henle is the portion of a nephron that leads from the proximal convoluted tubule to the distal convoluted tubule. It can be divided into two sections; the descending and the ascending loops (Figure 31.1). The thin descending limb has low permeability to ions and urea, while being highly permeable to water. The loop has a sharp bend in the renal medulla going from descending to ascending thin limb.

The thin ascending loop is impermeable to water, but it is permeable to ions. Sodium (Na^+), potassium (K^+) and chloride (Cl^-) ions are reabsorbed from the urine by secondary active transport by a Na-K-Cl cotransporter. The electrical and concentration gradient drives more reabsorption of Na^+, as well as other cations such as magnesium (Mg^{2+}) and calcium (Ca^{2+}).

The loop of Henle is supplied by blood in a series of straight capillaries descending from the cortical efferent arterioles. These capillaries (vasa recta) also have a counter-current multiplier mechanism that prevents washout of solutes from the medulla, thereby maintaining the medullary concentration. As water is osmotically moved from the descending limb into the interstitium, it readily enters the vasa recta. The low blood flow through the vasa recta allows time for osmotic equilibration, and can be altered by changing the resistance of the vessels' efferent arterioles.

Distal convoluted tubule

A distal convoluted tubule is a twisted, tube-like structure of the nephron (Figure 31.1). The distal convoluted tubule is the section farthest away from the renal corpuscle, and the cells that line it are able to actively pump potentially harmful substances, such as ammonia, urea and certain drugs, out of the blood and into the urine. From the distal convoluted tubule, useful substances are returned to the blood, while waste products and toxins are added to the filtrate. Hydrogen ions are also pumped in, making the urine pH more acidic. The distal convoluted tubule walls do not normally allow water to pass through, but the hormone ADH can open channels which allow water to move out, concentrating the urine.

Collecting ducts

From the distal convoluted tubule, filtrate drains into what are known as collecting ducts (Figure 31.1). These are tubes which receive filtrate from the distal convoluted tubules of many nephrons. Inside these collecting ducts, water can be absorbed to regulate the final concentration of urine produced by the kidneys. On leaving the collecting ducts, urine enters a space known as the renal pelvis, from where it passes into the bladder and is expelled from the body during urination.

The collecting duct system is under the control of ADH. In the absence of ADH, water in the renal filtrate is allowed to enter the urine, promoting diuresis. When ADH is present, aquaporins aid reabsorption of water, thereby inhibiting diuresis.

32 The kidney: macroscopic

Figure 32.1 External layers of the kidney

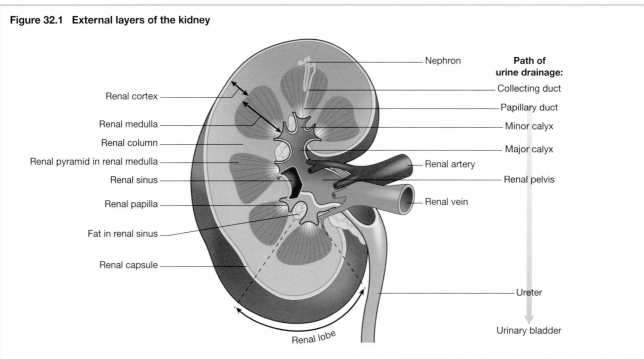

Nephron

Path of urine drainage:

Renal cortex

Collecting duct

Papillary duct

Renal medulla

Minor calyx

Renal column

Major calyx

Renal pyramid in renal medulla

Renal artery

Renal sinus

Renal pelvis

Renal papilla

Renal vein

Fat in renal sinus

Renal capsule

Ureter

Urinary bladder

Renal lobe

Source: Peate I, Wild K & Nair M (eds) Nursing Practice: Knowledge and Care (2014)

Figure 32.2 Blood flow through the kidney

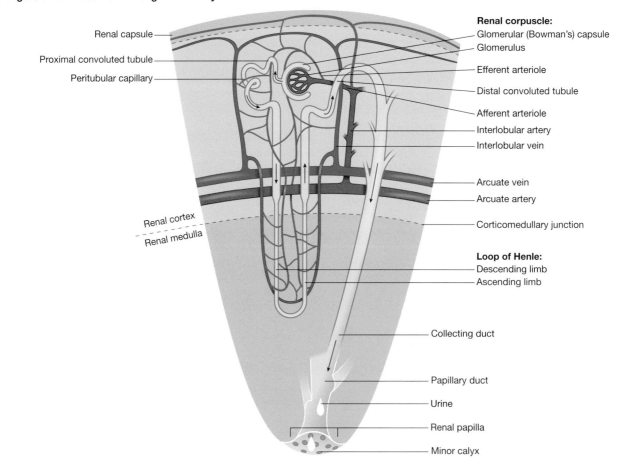

Renal capsule

Renal corpuscle:
Glomerular (Bowman's) capsule
Glomerulus

Proximal convoluted tubule

Efferent arteriole

Peritubular capillary

Distal convoluted tubule

Afferent arteriole

Interlobular artery

Interlobular vein

Arcuate vein

Arcuate artery

Renal cortex

Renal medulla

Corticomedullary junction

Loop of Henle:
Descending limb
Ascending limb

Collecting duct

Papillary duct

Urine

Renal papilla

Minor calyx

Anatomy and Physiology for Nurses at a Glance, First Edition. Ian Peate and Muralitharan Nair. © 2015 John Wiley & Sons, Ltd. Published 2015 by John Wiley & Sons, Ltd.
Companion website: www.ataglanceseries.com/nursing/anatomy

Kidney

There are two kidneys, one on each side of the spinal column. They are approximately 11 cm long, 5–6 cm wide and 3–4 cm thick. They are said to be bean-shaped organs where the outer border is convex; the inner border is known as the hilum (also known as hilus), and it is here that the renal arteries, renal veins, nerves and the ureters enter and leave the kidneys (Figure 32.1). The renal artery carries blood to the kidneys and once the blood is filtered the renal vein takes the blood away from the kidney. The right kidney is in contact with the liver's large right lobe and hence the right kidney is approximately 2–4 cm lower than the left kidney.

Each kidney is covered by three layers; the renal facia, adipose tissue and renal capsule. The real fascia is the outer layer and it consists of a thin layer of connective tissue that anchors the kidneys to the abdominal wall and the surrounding tissues. The middle layer is called the adipose tissue which surrounds the capsule. It cushions the kidneys from trauma. The inner layer is called the renal capsule. It consists of a layer of smooth connective tissue which is continuous of the outer layer of the ureter. The renal capsule protects the kidneys from trauma and maintains the shape of the kidneys.

Renal cortex

The renal cortex is the outer portion of the kidney between the renal capsule and the renal medulla. In the adult, it forms a continuous smooth outer zone with a number of projections (cortical columns) that extend down between the pyramids. It contains the renal corpuscles and the renal tubules except for parts of the loop of Henle which descend into the renal medulla. It also contains blood vessels and cortical collecting ducts.

Renal medulla

The renal medulla is a term used for the innermost portion of the kidney. The medulla is lighter in colour and has an abundance of blood vessels and tubules of the nephron. The renal medulla (pyramid) is composed of conical masses of tissue called renal pyramids, whose bases are directed toward the convex surface of the kidney, and which apex to form the renal papillae. The renal cortex forms a shell around the medulla. Its tissues dip into the medulla between adjacent renal pyramids to form renal columns. The granular appearance of the cortex is due to the random arrangement of tiny tubules associated with nephrons, the functional units of the kidney.

Renal pelvis

The renal pelvis forms the expanded upper portion of the ureter, which is funnel shaped, and it is the region where two or three calyces converge. These are cavities in which urine collects before it flows on into the urinary bladder. The renal pelvis is lined with a moist mucous-membrane layer that is only a few cells thick; the membrane is attached to a thicker coating of smooth muscle fibres, which, in turn, is surrounded by a layer of connective tissue. The mucous membrane of the pelvis is somewhat folded so that there is some room for tissue expansion when urine distends the pelvis.

The muscle fibres are arranged in a longitudinal and a circular layer. Contractions of the muscle layers occur in periodic waves known as peristaltic movements. The peristaltic waves help to push urine from the pelvis into the ureter and bladder. The lining of the pelvis and of the ureter is impermeable to the normal substances found in urine; thus, the walls of these structures do not absorb fluids.

Blood supply

The renal artery enters into the kidney at the level of first lumbar vertebra just below the superior mesenteric artery. The renal circulation receives approximately 20–25% of the cardiac output. It branches from the abdominal aorta and returns blood to the ascending vena cava. Each renal artery branches into segmental arteries, dividing further into interlobar arteries which penetrate the renal capsule and extend through the renal columns between the renal pyramids. The interlobar arteries then supply blood to the arcuate arteries that run through the boundary of the cortex and the medulla. Each arcuate artery supplies several interlobular arteries that feed into the afferent arterioles that supply the glomeruli (Figure 32.2).

From here, efferent arterioles leave the glomerulus and divide into peritubular capillaries, which drain into the interlobular veins and then into the arcuate vein and then into the interlobar vein, which runs into lobar vein, which opens into the segmental vein and which drains into the renal vein, and then from it blood moves into the inferior vena cava.

Nerve supply

The kidney and nervous system communicate via the renal plexus, whose fibres course along the renal arteries to reach each kidney. Input from the sympathetic nervous system triggers vasoconstriction in the kidney, thereby reducing renal blood flow. The kidney also receives input from the parasympathetic nervous system, by way of the renal branches of the Vagus nerve (Cranial nerve X). Sensory input from the kidney travels to the T10-11 levels of the spinal cord and is sensed in the corresponding dermatome.

33 The ureter, bladder and urethra

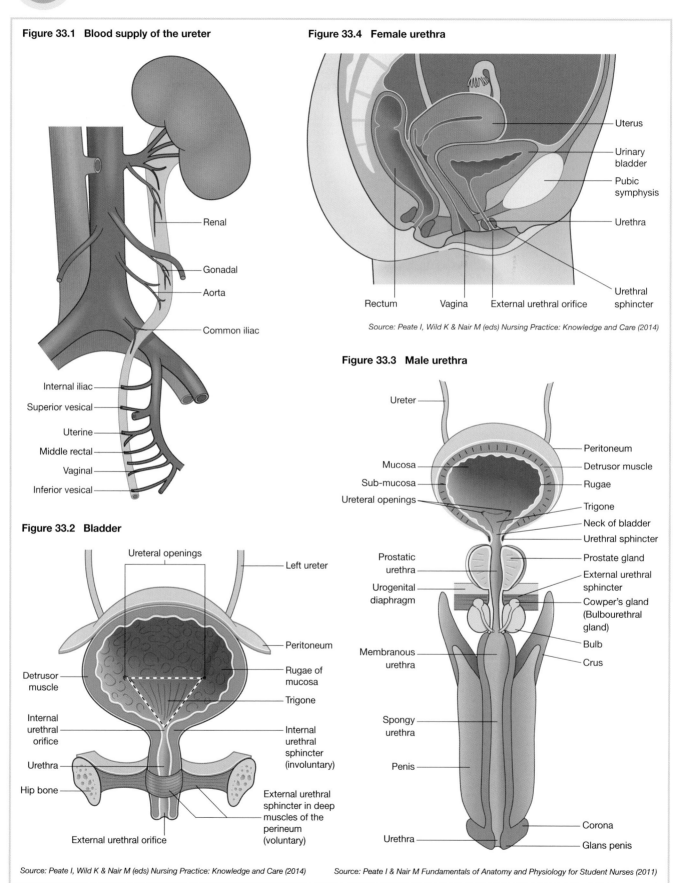

Figure 33.1 Blood supply of the ureter

Renal
Gonadal
Aorta
Common iliac
Internal iliac
Superior vesical
Uterine
Middle rectal
Vaginal
Inferior vesical

Figure 33.4 Female urethra

Uterus
Urinary bladder
Pubic symphysis
Urethra
Urethral sphincter
Rectum
Vagina
External urethral orifice

Source: Peate I, Wild K & Nair M (eds) Nursing Practice: Knowledge and Care (2014)

Figure 33.3 Male urethra

Ureter
Mucosa
Sub-mucosa
Ureteral openings
Prostatic urethra
Urogenital diaphragm
Membranous urethra
Spongy urethra
Penis
Urethra

Peritoneum
Detrusor muscle
Rugae
Trigone
Neck of bladder
Urethral sphincter
Prostate gland
External urethral sphincter
Cowper's gland (Bulbourethral gland)
Bulb
Crus
Corona
Glans penis

Figure 33.2 Bladder

Ureteral openings
Left ureter
Peritoneum
Rugae of mucosa
Trigone
Detrusor muscle
Internal urethral orifice
Urethra
Hip bone
External urethral orifice
Internal urethral sphincter (involuntary)
External urethral sphincter in deep muscles of the perineum (voluntary)

Source: Peate I, Wild K & Nair M (eds) Nursing Practice: Knowledge and Care (2014)

Source: Peate I & Nair M Fundamentals of Anatomy and Physiology for Student Nurses (2011)

Anatomy and Physiology for Nurses at a Glance, First Edition. Ian Peate and Muralitharan Nair. © 2015 John Wiley & Sons, Ltd. Published 2015 by John Wiley & Sons, Ltd.
Companion website: www.ataglanceseries.com/nursing/anatomy

Ureters

The ureters transport urine from the pelvis of the kidney to the bladder. The flow of urine is as a result of peristaltic contraction of the muscular walls of the ureter. Approximately 1–5 peristaltic waves form every minute depending on the formation of urine.

Abdominal ureter

The ureter is roughly 25–30 cm long in adults and courses down the retroperitoneum in an S curve. At the proximal end of the ureter is the renal pelvis; at the distal end is the bladder. The ureter begins at the level of the renal artery and vein posterior to these structures.

Pelvic ureter

The ureter enters the pelvis, where it crosses anteriorly to the iliac vessels, which usually occurs at the bifurcation of the common iliac artery into the internal and external iliac arteries. Here, the ureters are within 5 cm of one another before they diverge laterally.

Blood supply

The vascular supply and venous drainage of the ureter is derived from varied and numerous vessels. In the abdominal ureter, the arterial supply is located on the medial aspect of the ureter, whereas in the pelvis, the lateral aspect is the area for the blood supply (Figure 33.1).

Urinary bladder

The urinary bladder is a hollow muscular organ and is located in the pelvic cavity posterior to the symphysis pubis. In the male the bladder lies anterior to the rectum and in the female it lies anterior to the vagina and inferior to the uterus; it is a smooth muscular sac which stores urine. When the bladder is empty, the inner section of the bladder forms folds but as the bladder fills up with urine the walls of the bladder become smoother (Figure 33.2). The bladder normally distends and holds approximately 300–350 ml of urine. In females the bladder is slightly smaller because the uterus occupies the space above the bladder.

Layers of the bladder

The bladder is composed of three layers. The serous coat (tunica serosa) is a partial one, and is derived from the peritoneum. The muscular coat (tunica muscularis) consists of three layers of unstriped muscular fibres: an external layer composed of fibres having for the most part a longitudinal arrangement; a middle layer, in which the fibres are arranged, more or less, in a circular manner; and an internal layer, in which the fibres have a general longitudinal arrangement. The mucous coat (tunica mucosa) is thin, smooth and of a pale rose colour. It is continuous above through the ureters with the lining membrane of the renal tubules, and below with that of the urethra.

Vessels and nerves

The arteries supplying the bladder are the superior, middle and inferior vesical, derived from the anterior trunk of the hypogastric. The obturator and inferior gluteal arteries also supply small visceral branches to the bladder, and in the female additional branches are derived from the uterine and vaginal arteries.

The nerves of the bladder are (i) fine medullated fibres from the third and fourth sacral nerves, and (ii) non-medullated fibres from the hypogastric plexus.

Urethra

The urethra is a muscular tube that drains urine from the bladder and conveys it out of the body. It contains three coats and they are muscular, erectile and mucous, the muscular is the continuation of the bladder muscle layer. The urethra is encompassed by two separate urethral sphincter muscles. The internal urethral sphincter muscle is formed by involuntary smooth muscles while the lower voluntary muscles make up the external sphincter muscles. The internal sphincter is created by the detrusor muscle. Sphincters keep the urethra closed when urine is not being passed. The internal urethral sphincter is under involuntary control and lies at the bladder–urethra junction. The external urethral sphincter is under voluntary control.

Male urethra

In the male, the urethra not only excretes fluid wastes but is also part of the reproductive system. Rather than the straight tube found in the female body, the male urethra is shaped like a 'S' to follow the line of the penis. It is approximately 20 centimetres long (Figure 33.3). The male urethra passes through three regions: prostatic, membranous (shortest and least distensible portion of the urethra) and the penile urethra (is the region that spans the corpus spongiosum of the penis).

The prostatic portion is only about 2.5 cm long and passes along the neck of the urinary bladder through the prostate gland. This section is designed to accept the drainage from the tiny ducts within the prostate and is equipped with two ejaculatory tubes.

Female urethra

The female urethra is bound to the anterior vaginal wall. The external opening of the urethra is anterior to the vagina and posterior to the clitoris. In the female, the urethra is approximately 4 centimetres long and leads out of the body via urethral orifice. In the female, the urethral orifice is located in the vestibule in the labia minora. This can be found located in between the clitoris and the vaginal orifice (Figure 33.4). In the female body the urethra's only function is to transport urine out of the body.

34 Formation of urine

Figure 34.1 Renal filtration

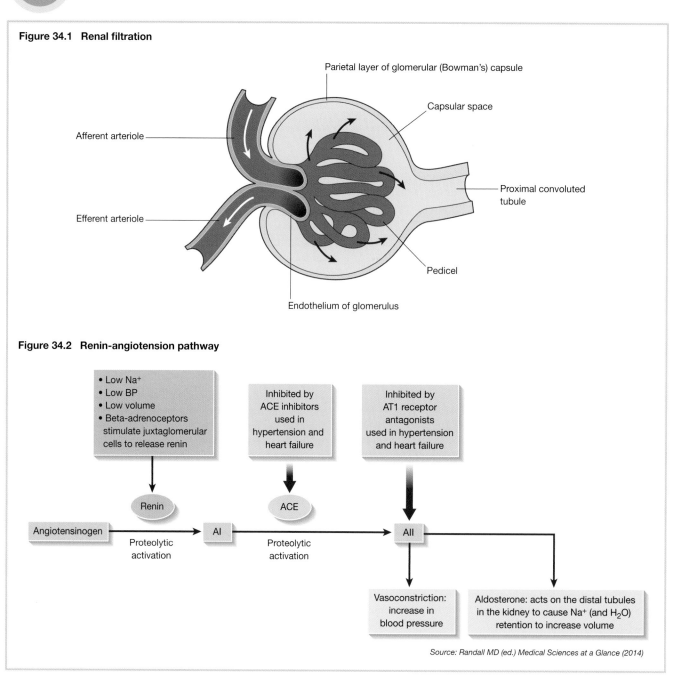

Figure 34.2 Renin-angiotension pathway

Source: Randall MD (ed.) Medical Sciences at a Glance (2014)

Three processes are involved in the formation of urine and they are filtration, selective reabsorption and secretion.

Filtration

Urine formation begins with the process of filtration of the blood, which goes on continually in the renal corpuscles. As blood passes through the glomeruli, much of its fluid, containing both useful chemicals and dissolved waste materials, flows out of the blood through the membranes (by osmosis and diffusion) where it is filtered and then flows into the Bowman's capsule. This process is called glomerular filtration (Figure 34.1). The water, waste products, salt, glucose and other chemicals that have been filtered out of the blood are known collectively as glomerular filtrate. The glomerular filtrate consists primarily of water, excess salts (sodium and potassium), glucose, and a waste product of the body called urea. Urea is formed in the body to eliminate the very toxic ammonia products that are formed in the liver from amino acids. Since humans cannot excrete ammonia, it is converted to the less dangerous urea and then filtered out of the blood. Urea is the most abundant of the waste products that must be excreted by the kidneys.

Selective reabsorption

The PCT has a microvilli cell border to increase the surface area for absorption from filtrate. There are also a large number of mitochondria which produce the extra ATP required for active transport. Substances reabsorbed back into the blood stream are water, glucose and other nutrients, and sodium (Na^+) and other ions. Reabsorption begins in the proximal convoluted tubules and continues in the loop of Henle, distal convoluted tubules, and collecting tubules. Only 1% of the glomerular filtrate actually leaves the body and 99% is reabsorbed back into the blood stream.

Blood glucose is entirely reabsorbed back into the blood from the proximal tubules. In fact, it is actively transported out of the tubules and into the peritubular capillary blood. None of this valuable nutrient is wasted by being lost in the urine.

Other components, such as ammonia and urea, are secreted rather than absorbed, while certain ions, including potassium, can be both secreted and absorbed by the tubules according to the overall ionic balance throughout the body.

Secretion

Any substances not removed through filtration are secreted into the renal tubules from the peritubular capillaries of the nephron, these include drugs and hydrogen ions. Tubular secretion mainly takes place by active transport system. Active transport is a process by which substances are moved across biological membrane. Tubular secretion occurs from epithelial cells lining the renal tubules and the collecting ducts.

Substances secreted are hydrogen ions (H^+), potassium ions (K^+), ammonia (NH_3) and certain drugs. Kidney tubule secretion plays a crucial role in maintaining the body's acid-base balance, another example of an important body function that the kidney participates in.

Hormonal control

Four hormones play a role in the regulation of fluid and electrolytes and they are ADH, angiotensin, aldosterone and atrial natriuretic peptide.

ADH

ADH is produced by the hypothalamus gland and is stored by the posterior pituitary gland. This hormone increases the permeability of the cells in the distal convoluted tubule and the collecting ducts. In the presence of ADH more water is reabsorbed from the renal tubules and therefore the patient will pass less urine. In the absence of ADH less water is reabsorbed and the patient will pass more urine. Thus ADH plays a major role in the regulation of fluid balance in the body.

Angiotension

Renin-angiotensin is a hormone system that regulates blood pressure and water (fluid) balance. When blood volume is low, juxtaglomerular cells in the kidneys secrete renin directly into circulation. Plasma renin then carries out the conversion of angiotensinogen released by the liver to angiotensin I. Angiotensin I is subsequently converted to angiotensin II by the angiotensin converting enzyme found in the lungs. Angiotensin II is a potent vaso-active peptide that causes blood vessels to constrict, resulting in increased blood pressure. Angiotensin II also stimulates the secretion of the hormone aldosterone from the adrenal cortex. Aldosterone causes the tubules of the kidneys to increase the reabsorption of sodium and water into the blood. This increases the volume of fluid in the body, which also increases blood pressure (Figure 34.2).

Aldosterone

A steroid hormone secreted by the adrenal glands. Aldosterone serves as the principal regulator of the salt and water balance of the body and thus is categorised as a mineralocorticoid. It also has a small effect on the metabolism of fats, carbohydrates and proteins.

Several things will stimulate aldosterone secretion: when the potassium levels go too high, if there is less blood flow to the kidneys, or if the blood pressure falls. The converse is aldosterone secretion will decrease if the potassium levels fall, the blood flow in the kidneys increases, blood volume increases or if one consumes too much salt.

Atrial natriuretic peptide (ANP)

This is a peptide hormone secreted by myocytes of the cardiac atria that promotes salt and water excretion and lowers blood pressure. ANP acts to reduce the water, sodium and adipose loads on the circulatory system, thereby reducing blood pressure. ANP has exactly the opposite function of the aldosterone secreted by the zona glomerulosa. Synthesis of ANP also takes place in the ventricles, brain, suprarenal glands and renal glands. It is released in response to atrial stretch.

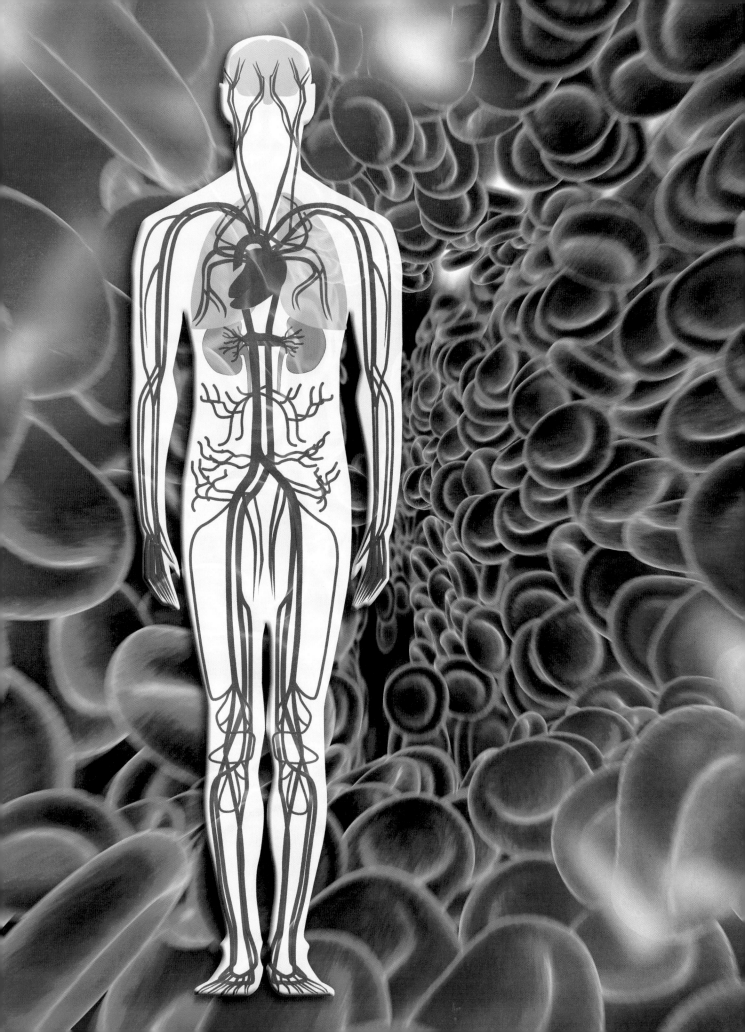

The male reproductive system

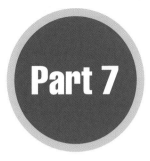

Part 7

Chapters

35 External male genitalia

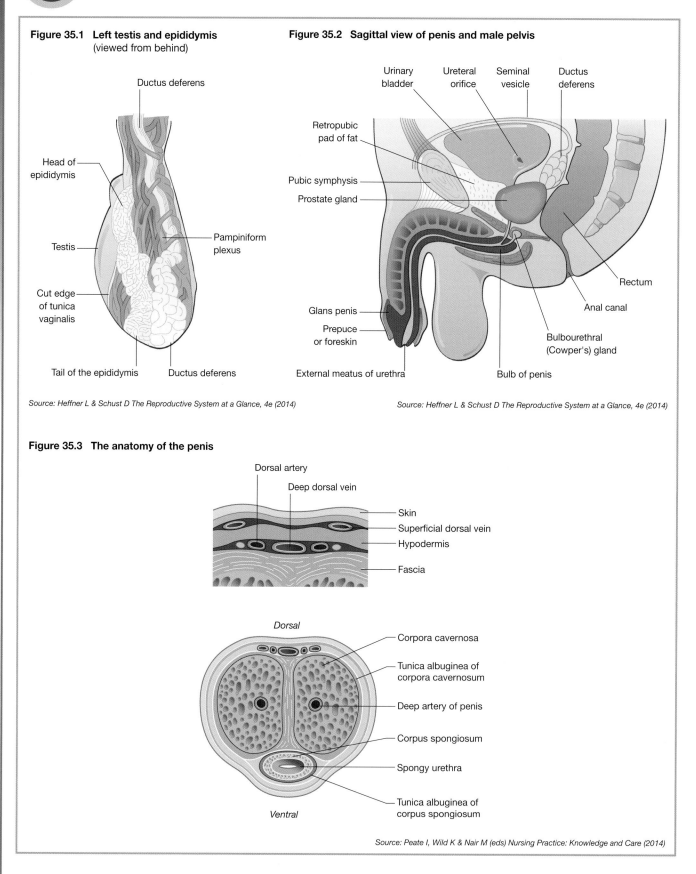

Figure 35.1 Left testis and epididymis
(viewed from behind)

Ductus deferens

Head of
epididymis

Testis

Pampiniform
plexus

Cut edge
of tunica
vaginalis

Tail of the epididymis

Ductus deferens

Source: Heffner L & Schust D The Reproductive System at a Glance, 4e (2014)

Figure 35.2 Sagittal view of penis and male pelvis

Urinary
bladder

Ureteral
orifice

Seminal
vesicle

Ductus
deferens

Retropubic
pad of fat

Pubic symphysis

Prostate gland

Glans penis

Prepuce
or foreskin

External meatus of urethra

Rectum

Anal canal

Bulbourethral
(Cowper's) gland

Bulb of penis

Source: Heffner L & Schust D The Reproductive System at a Glance, 4e (2014)

Figure 35.3 The anatomy of the penis

Dorsal artery

Deep dorsal vein

Skin

Superficial dorsal vein

Hypodermis

Fascia

Dorsal

Corpora cavernosa

Tunica albuginea of
corpora cavernosum

Deep artery of penis

Corpus spongiosum

Spongy urethra

Tunica albuginea of
corpus spongiosum

Ventral

Source: Peate I, Wild K & Nair M (eds) Nursing Practice: Knowledge and Care (2014)

Unlike the female reproductive system the male reproductive system is more evident as the majority of the organs of the male reproductive system are located externally (see Figure 35.1 and 35.2). The prostate gland is discussed in Chapter 36.

The male reproductive system works with other body systems, producing hormones essential for biological development, sexual behaviour and sexual performance. Other body systems include the neuroendocrine system and the musculoskeletal system. The male reproductive system is also central to the function of the urinary system.

The male reproductive system includes the scrotum, testes, spermatic ducts, sex glands and the penis. Working together these organs produce sperm, the male gamete and the other components of semen. These organs also work together to deliver semen out of the body and into the vagina where it can fertilise egg cells in order to reproduce.

The key functions of the male reproductive system are to:
• Produce, maintain and transport the male reproductive cells (sperm) as well as the fluid semen.
• To ejaculate semen from the penis.
• To produce and secrete the male sex hormones.

The testes

The reproductive glands of the male are the testes, these are the male equivalent to the ovaries.

Developmentally the testes are located in the abdominal cavity of the foetus, descending down through the inguinal canal into the scrotal sac, suspended on either side of the penis, it is usual for one to hang lower than the other. The testes are external to the body. For sperm to be sustainable it must be produced at a temperature lower than core body temperature, this is why the testes are located in the scrotal sac external to the body.

The testes are oval shaped organs approximately the size of very large olives lying in the scrotal sac, secured and suspendered at either end of the spermatic cord. There are usually two testes. Three layers of serous fibrous tissue, the tunica vaginalis, the tunica albuginea and the tunica vasculosa surround them.

The testes are responsible for producing testosterone, the primary male sex hormone, they also generate sperm. Within the testes are coiled masses of tubes – seminiferous tubules. These are responsible for producing the sperm cells through spermatogenesis. There are spaces between the tubules comprising a cluster of cells – Leydig cells that have the responsibility to manufacture and secrete testosterone and other androgens.

Spermatogenesis

Spermatogenesis occurs in the seminiferous tubules of the testes and usually begins around puberty. Starting at puberty, a male will produce millions of sperm every single day for the rest of his life. The seminiferous tubules contain diploid cells – spermatogonium that mature to become sperm. Spermatogenesis turns each one of the diploid spermatogonium into four haploid sperm cells, quadrupling is accomplished through the meiotic cell division.

During interphase before meiosis I, the spermatogonium's 46 single chromosomes are duplicated to form 46 pairs of sister chromatids, these exchange genetic material through synapsis before the first meiotic division. In meiosis II, the two daughter cells divide again producing four cells containing a unique set of 23 single chromosomes that eventually develop into four sperm cells. The sperm are released from the Sertoli cells entering the lumen of the seminiferous tubules and are pushed along the various ducts within the testes.

The penis

The penis is the male organ for sexual intercourse. It has three parts: the root, attached to the wall of the abdomen; the body, or shaft and the glans at the end of the penis. The glans, (when present), is covered with a loose layer of skin, the foreskin. The opening of the urethra transports semen and urine, at the tip of the glans penis. The penis contains a number of sensitive nerve endings and is highly vascular.

The body is cylindrical consisting of three internal chambers, they are made up of special, sponge-like erectile tissue, containing thousands of large spaces that fill with blood when sexually aroused (see Figure 35.3). As it fills with blood, it becomes rigid and erect, allowing for sexual penetration. Penile skin is loose and elastic accommodating changes in penis size during an erection. When the penile compartments fill with blood, parasympathetic nervous system arteriolar vasodilation takes occurs. The erection reflex is prompted by sight, sound, smell, touch, pressure or visual stimulation. After ejaculation vasoconstriction of the arterioles occurs and the penis become flaccid

The epididymis

The epididymis is a long, coiled tube that rests on the backside of each testicle, transporting and storing sperm cells produced in the testes. The epididymis brings sperm to maturity, as sperm leaving the testes are immature, and are unable to fertilise the egg.

The vas deferens, ejaculatory ducts and spermatic cord

The vas deferens is a long, muscular tube travelling from the epididymis into the pelvic cavity behind the bladder, transporting mature sperm to the urethra ready for ejaculation. The ejaculatory ducts formed by the fusion of the vas deferens and the seminal vesicles empty into the urethra. In the male the urethra carries urine from the bladder to outside of the body and expels semen during orgasm. The seminal vesicles are sac-like pouches attached to the vas deferens near the base of the bladder producing a fructose-rich fluid providing sperm with a source of energy and assisting with motility.

36 The prostate gland

Figure 36.1   The zones of the prostate gland

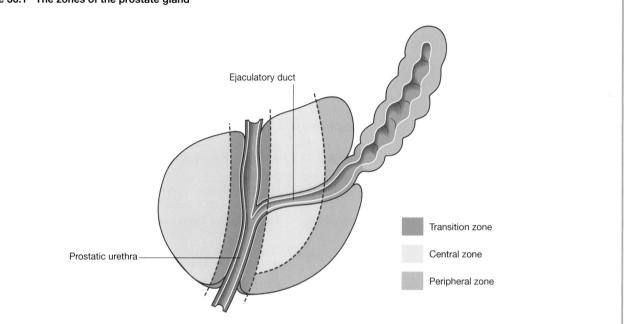

Ejaculatory duct

Prostatic urethra

Transition zone

Central zone

Peripheral zone

Anatomy and Physiology for Nurses at a Glance, First Edition. Ian Peate and Muralitharan Nair. © 2015 John Wiley & Sons, Ltd. Published 2015 by John Wiley & Sons, Ltd.
Companion website: www.ataglanceseries.com/nursing/anatomy

Not all of the functions of the prostate gland are well understood; the prostate is an exocrine gland and part of the male reproductive system

The gland

The prostate is covered in a layer of fibrous tissue called the prostatic capsule. There is a thin layer of connective tissue that separates the prostate and seminal vesicles from the rectum posteriorly.

The prostate gland is made up of different types of cells:
- gland cells that produce the fluid portion of semen
- muscle cells that control urine flow and ejaculation
- fibrous cells that provide the supportive structure of the gland

The prostate gland is firm, it is partly glandular and has a partly muscular body, located immediately below the internal urethral orifice and around the beginning of the urethra. It is found in the pelvic cavity, below the lower part of the symphysis pubis, above the superior fascia of the urogenital diaphragm and in front of the rectum. It is about the size of a chestnut and somewhat conical in shape with three zones (see Figure 36.1).

Arterial supply to the prostate is derived from branches of the internal iliac artery, venous blood collects in the periprostatic venous plexus where it is returned to the internal iliac vein by the inferior vesical vein.

Lymphatics from the prostate typically travel to internal iliac nodes, including the more anterior group of obturator nodes.

The prostate receives autonomic nerve supply from the inferior hypogastric plexus, which lies along the internal iliac artery.

The zones of the prostate gland
The peripheral zone

The peripheral zone is the area of the prostate that is closest to the rectum. It is the largest zone of the prostate gland and accounts for 70% of the total gland.

The transition zone

The transition zone is the middle area of the prostate, located between the peripheral and central zones. It surrounds the urethra as it passes through the prostate. Up until the age of 40 years this zone makes up approximately 20% of the prostate gland. As a man ages, the transition zone begins to enlarge, until it becomes the largest area of the prostate. As the transition zone enlarges, it then pushes the peripheral zone of the prostate toward the rectum.

Central zone

The central zone is in front of the transition zone. This zone is farthest from the rectum and contains approximately 1/3 of the ducts that secrete fluid that helps create semen.

The gland has a number of surfaces: a base, an apex, an anterior, a posterior and two lateral surfaces.

The surfaces of the prostate gland
The base

The base on palpation is directed upwards and inferior to the surface of the bladder. The urethra penetrates it closer to its anterior border than its posterior border.

The apex

The apex is small and is directed downwards and in contact with the urogenital diaphragm. The urethra exits through the apex.

The anterior, inferolateral and posterior surfaces

The anterior surface is narrow and is connected with the puboprostatic ligament. The paired inferolateral surfaces, which are separated from the levatores ani by the prostatic venous plexus, curve inwards both anteriorly and inferiorly. The posterior surface is broad, narrows inferiorly and can be defined by a shallow longitudinal depression into the right and left sides. The ejaculatory ducts join the prostate near the superior extent of this ridge.

The function of the prostate gland
Prostatic fluid

The key function of the prostate gland (which is regulated by the hormone testosterone) is to produce the fluid aspect of semen, this assists with motility and survival by providing a protective and fluid medium for the passage of semen through the vagina for fertilisation, this is an alkaline fluid. The gland cells within the prostate produce a thin fluid that is rich in proteins and minerals that maintain and nourish the sperm. This fluid is continually produced but when the man is sexually aroused, the prostate produces larger amounts of prostatic fluid. It then mixes with sperm and this is then ejaculated as semen.

The prostate also controls the flow of urine. The muscle fibres of the gland are wrapped around the urethra under involuntary nervous system control. These fibres contract to slow and stop the flow of urine.

Some structures around the prostate

- Seminal vesicles – These glands produce semen and are located on both sides of the prostate.
- Vas deferens – These tubes carry sperm from the testicles to the seminal vesicles.
- Nerve bundles – These nerves control bladder and erectile function and are found on both sides of the prostate.
- Muscles – These muscles control urination.

Prostate-specific antigen (PSA)

This is a fluid that is produced in the prostate playing a key role in enabling sperm to travel into the uterus by preserving the semen in liquid form. PSA is produced exclusively by epithelial prostatic cells. It counteracts the clotting enzyme in the seminal vesicle fluid, which principally glues the semen to the cervix, located next to the uterine entrance inside the vagina. PSA dissolves this enzyme with its own enzyme in order to permit the sperm to enter the uterus and impregnate an egg.

37 Spermatogenesis

Figure 37.1 Spermatogenesis

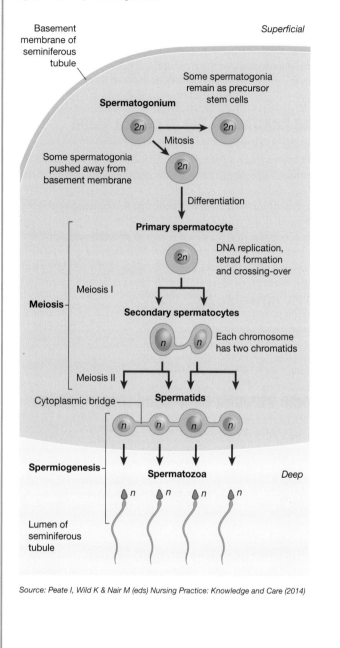

Basement membrane of seminiferous tubule

Superficial

Some spermatogonia remain as precursor stem cells

Spermatogonium

2n → 2n

Mitosis

Some spermatogonia pushed away from basement membrane

2n

Differentiation

Primary spermatocyte

2n

DNA replication, tetrad formation and crossing-over

Meiosis I

Meiosis

Secondary spermatocytes

n   n

Each chromosome has two chromatids

Meiosis II

Cytoplasmic bridge

Spermatids

n   n   n   n

Spermiogenesis

Spermatozoa

Deep

n   n   n   n

Lumen of seminiferous tubule

Source: Peate I, Wild K & Nair M (eds) Nursing Practice: Knowledge and Care (2014)

Figure 37.2 Primary and secondary sex characteristics

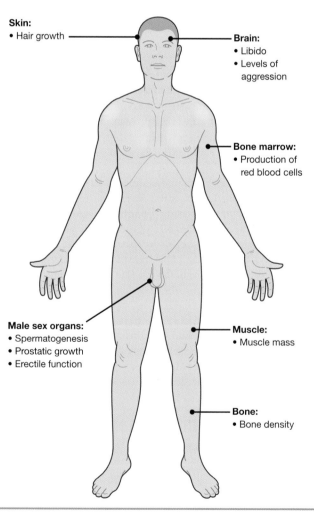

Skin:
• Hair growth

Brain:
• Libido
• Levels of aggression

Bone marrow:
• Production of red blood cells

Male sex organs:
• Spermatogenesis
• Prostatic growth
• Erectile function

Muscle:
• Muscle mass

Bone:
• Bone density

The process by which the spermatogonia (the male primordial germ cell) undergo meiosis producing a number of spermatozoa is called spermatogenesis. This process commences at puberty, continuing for as long as the man lives, as opposed to oogenesis (the production of the primordial ova), which occurs only during foetal life.

Spermatogenesis

The process by which male primary sperm cells undergo meiosis is called spermatogenesis and results in the production of a number of cells termed spermatogonia, from which the primary spermatocytes are derived. Each primary spermatocyte divides into two secondary spermatocytes; and each secondary spermatocyte into two spermatids or young spermatozoa. These develop into mature spermatozoa, also known as sperm cells. The primary spermatocyte gives rise to two cells, the secondary spermatocytes; and the two secondary spermatocytes, by their subdivision, produce four spermatozoa.

Spermatogenesis occurs in the seminiferous tubules of the testes (see Figure 37.1). Diploid (46 chromosome) germ cells known as spermatogonia line the basement membrane of each seminiferous tubule. The spermatogonia move away from the basement membrane as meiosis occurs, as they mature they become primary spermatocytes. Meiosis occurs again and this produces two haploid (23 chromosome) cells called secondary spermatocytes. Four spermatids are the result of the two secondary spermatocytes undergoing meiosis.

For spermatids to develop into sperm this is dependent on the Sertoli cells that are present in the seminiferous tubules. Attaching themselves to the Sertoli cells the spermatids receive the nourishment needed and the hormonal signals required to develop into sperm.

It has been estimated to take approximately 70 to 80 days for spermatogenesis to occur – from meiotic division of spermatogonium to the maturation of a mature spermatid. The mature sperm travel from the seminiferous tubules to the epididymis, their capacity for fertilisation continues to occur. Whilst the sperm are fully matured by the time they are ejaculated they do not become motile until they are activated by the action of biochemicals in the semen and in the female reproductive tract.

Semen is a white or grey liquid that is discharged from the urethra on ejaculation. Usually, each millilitre of semen contains millions of spermatozoa, but the majority of the volume is made up of secretions of the glands in the male reproductive organs.

Sperm will only survive in warm environments, as the sperm leave the body the sperm's survival is reduced and this may cause the cell to die, this decreases the quality of the sperm. There are two types of sperm cells 'male' and 'female'. Those sperm cells that give rise to female (XX) offspring after fertilization differ in so far as they carry an X chromosome, while sperm cells that give rise to male (XY) offspring only carry a Y chromosome.

The sperm cell is made up of a head, a midpiece and a tail. The head contains the nucleus containing densely coiled chromatin fibres, surrounded anteriorly by an acrosome, which contains enzymes that are used for penetrating the female egg. The midpiece has a central filamentous core with a number of mitochondria spiralled around it, used for adenosine triphosphate (ATP) production required for the journey through the female cervix, uterus and uterine tubes. The tail or 'flagellum' performs the lashing movements that are needed to propel the spermatocyte.

Male sex hormones

The major female and male hormones can be classified as oestrogens or androgens. Both classes of male and female hormones are present in both males and females alike, however they differ vastly in their amounts. Testosterone is the primary male sex hormone; it is a steroid that regulates growth and development.

Testosterone production increases exponentially (approximately 18-fold) during puberty. It is usual after puberty for the interstitial cells to produce testosterone continually. Approximately 6 mg of testosterone is produced each day. Testosterone production may be disrupted for a number of reasons. Once a man reaches 40 years of age testosterone production declines, on average men experience a 1% per year drop in testosterone production once they reach this age.

Testosterone functions to develop a man's primary and secondary sex characteristics (see Figure 37.2). Primary sex characteristics include size of penis and testes size in adult men – testosterone is responsible for developing the male genitals, spermatogenesis, and regulating the libido. Erectile function is influenced by testosterone as this increases the activity of nitric oxide synthase which regulates the movement of smooth muscles in the penis. Increased nitric oxide synthase activity increases relaxation of smooth muscles in the penis improving the ability to achieve and maintain an erection.

Secondary sex characteristics include the growth of hair (pubic, body and facial hair), a deep voice and heavier bones. Greater quantities of testosterone cause men to have a greater proportion of lean body mass and lower proportion of fat compared to women.

When the male reaches puberty there is an increase in the secretion of gonadotrophin-releasing hormone (GnRH) from the hypothalamus. GnRH then stimulates the anterior aspect of the pituitary gland to increase secretion of luteinising hormone (LH) and follicle stimulating hormone (FSH), this negative feedback mechanism controls secretion of testosterone and spermatogenesis.

The Leydig cells (located between seminiferous tubules) are stimulated by LH to secrete testosterone, testosterone is synthesised from cholesterol in the testes. The Leydig cells produce 95% of a man's testosterone. Through negative feedback the secretion of LH is suppressed by the anterior pituitary as well as suppressed secretion of GnRH by the hypothalamus. Testosterone in some target cells, for example in the prostate gland, is converted to dihydrotestosterone (DHT).

FSH indirectly acts to stimulate spermatogenesis with FSH and testosterone acting synergistically on the Sertoli cells to stimulate discharge of androgen-binding protein (ABP) into the lumen of the seminiferous tubules as well as the interstitial fluid surrounding the spermatogenic cells. ABP attaches to testosterone keeping the concentration high. Testosterone is responsible for stimulating the final steps of spermatogenesis in the seminiferous tubules.

Sertoli cells release inhibin once the degree of spermatogenesis required for male reproduction functions has been achieved, inhibin (a hormone) inhibits FSH secretion by the anterior pituitary gland, less inhibin is released when spermatogenesis is happening too slowly and as such more FHS is produced, resulting in an increased rate of spermatogenesis.

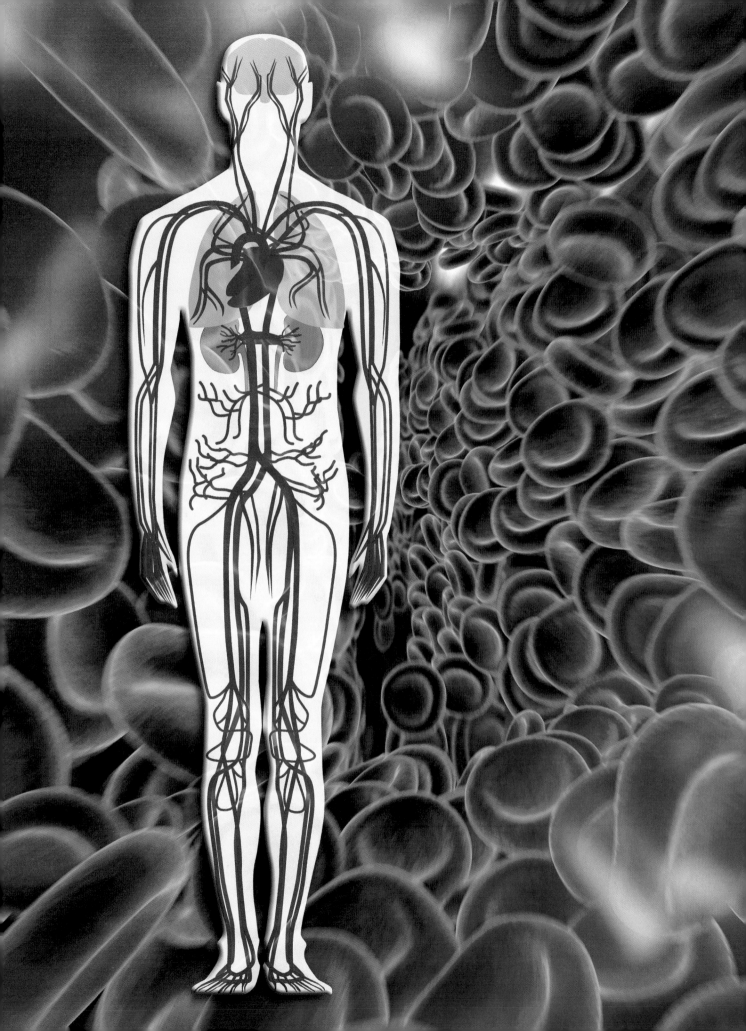

The female reproductive system

Part 8

Chapters

Female internal reproductive organs

Figure 38.1 The female internal reproductive organs

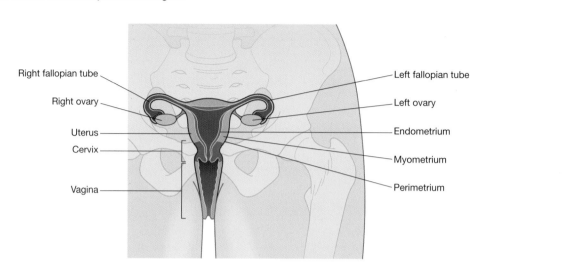

Right fallopian tube

Right ovary

Uterus

Cervix

Vagina

Left fallopian tube

Left ovary

Endometrium

Myometrium

Perimetrium

Table 38.1 The layers of the uterus

Layer	Comments
The perimetrium	A serous membrane that envelopes the uterus, the outer layer; provides support to the uterus located within the pelvis. Also known as the parietal peritoneum.
The myometrium	The middle layer made up of smooth muscle. Throughout pregnancy and childbirth the uterus has to stretch and the muscular layer permits this to occur. The muscle will contact during labour and post natally this muscular layer contracts forcefully to force out the placenta.
The endometrium	The inner layer of the uterus with a mucus lining. The exterior is continuous with the vagina and the fallopian tubes. During menstruation the layers of the endometrium are shed, sloughing away from the inner layer, this is the menstrual period occurring as a result of hormonal changes taking place. The endometrium thickens during the menstrual period becoming rich with blood vessels and glandular tissue until the next period occurs and the cycle begins again.

Anatomy and Physiology for Nurses at a Glance, First Edition. Ian Peate and Muralitharan Nair. © 2015 John Wiley & Sons, Ltd. Published 2015 by John Wiley & Sons, Ltd.
Companion website: www.ataglanceseries.com/nursing/anatomy

The female reproduction system produces the female egg cells (ova or oocytes) essential for reproduction and the female sex hormones that maintain the reproductive cycle. This system is both a reproductive system as well as containing the female sex organs.

The internal female reproductive organs

The female internal sex organs consist of the ovaries, the fallopian tubes, the uterus and the vagina (see Figure 38.1).

The ovaries

The ovaries are the primary reproductive organs as well as producing female sex hormones; they are paired glands, in the adult woman they are flat, almond-shaped structures situated on each side of the uterus beneath the ends of the fallopian tubes. Ligaments hold them in position attaching them to the uterus; they are also attached to the broad ligament, this ligament attaches them to the pelvic wall. The ovaries provide a space for storage of the female germ cells and also produce the female hormones oestrogen and progesterone. A woman's total number of ova is present at her birth, when a girl reaches puberty she usually ovulates each month.

The ovary contains a number of small structures, these are called ovarian follicles. Each follicle contains an immature ovum, (an oocyte). Follicles are stimulated each month by two hormones – the follicle-stimulating hormone (FSH) and luteinising hormone (LH) – these stimulate the follicles to mature. The developing follicles are enclosed in layers of follicle cells, mature follicles are called graafian follicles.

The ovarian cortex

This lies deep and close to the tunica albuginea containing the ovarian follicles surrounded by dense irregular connective tissue. These follicles contain oocytes in different stages of development and a number of cells that feed the developing oocyte, as the follicle grows it secretes oestrogen.

Graafian follicles

The graafian follicles manufacture oestrogen, stimulating the growth of endometrium. Each month in the woman who is menstruating, one or two of the mature follicles (the graafian follicles) release an oocyte in what is known as ovulation. The large ruptured follicle becomes a new structure – the corpus luteum, the remnants of a mature follicle.

Corpus luteum

The corpus luteum produces oestrogen and progesterone to support the endometrium until conception or the cycle begins again. The corpus luteum gradually disintegrates; a scar is left on the outside of the ovary (the corpus albicans). The outer ovary is enveloped in a fibrous capsule called the tunica albuginea, this is composed of cuboidal epithelium. The inner ovary is divided into parts.

The ovarian medulla

The ovarian medulla contains blood vessels, nerves and lymphatic tissues surrounded by loose connective tissue.

Oogenesis

This relates to the development of relatively undifferentiated germ cells – oogonia – which are fixed to between 2 to 4 million diploid (2n) stem cells during foetal development. All ova are ultimately derived from these clones as they develop into larger primary oocytes, the meiotic phase is not completed until puberty.

Every month after puberty until menopause, FSH and LH are released by the anterior pituitary gland stimulating primordial follicles, only one usually reaches the maturity needed for ovulation.

Female sex hormones

The ovaries produce oestrogens, progesterone and androgens recurrently.

Oestrogens are essential for the development and maintenance of secondary sex characteristics working with a number of other hormones, stimulating the female reproductive organ to prepare for the growth of a foetus, playing a key role in the usual structure of the skin and blood vessels. They help reduce the rate of bone resorption, enhance increased high-density lipoproteins, decrease cholesterol levels and increase blood clotting.

The uterus

A hollow muscular organ in the pelvic cavity posterior and superior to the urinary bladder, anterior to the rectum, approximately 7.5 cm long. The fundus is a thick muscular region above the fallopian tubes; the body is joined to the cervix by the isthmus. The uterus also has three layers; the uterine wall has three distinct layers (see Table 38.1).

The fallopian tubes

The paired fallopian tubes are delicate, thin cylindrical structures approximately 8–14 cm long, affixed to the uterus on one end supported by the broad ligaments. The lateral ends of the fallopian tubes are open and made of projections called fimbriae draped over the ovary. The fimbriae pick up the ovum after discharge from the ovary; they are composed of smooth muscle lined with ciliated mucous-producing epithelial cells, transporting the ovum along the tubes towards the uterus. Fertilisation of the ovum usually occurs in the outer portion of the fallopian tubes.

The vagina

A tubular, fibromuscular structure approximately 8 to 10 cm in length, it is the receptacle for the penis during sexual intercourse, an organ of sexual response, the canal allows the menstrual flow to leave the body and is the passage for the birth of the child. It is situated posterior to the urinary bladder and urethra, anterior to the rectum. The upper element houses the uterine cervix. Vaginal walls are made of membranous folds of rugae, composed of mucous-secreting stratified squamous epithelial cells.

Usually the vaginal walls are moist with a pH ranging from 3.8 to 4.2. Oestrogen causes the growth of vaginal mucosal cells, thickening and developing them, increasing glycogen content resulting in a slight acidifying of the vaginal fluid.

The cervix

The cervix forms a pathway between the uterus and the vagina. The uterine opening of the cervix is the internal os and the vaginal opening the external os. The space between these openings, the endocervical canal, acts as a conduit for the discharge of menstrual fluid, the opening for sperm and delivery of the infant during birth.

39 External female genitalia

Figure 39.1 The female external genitalia

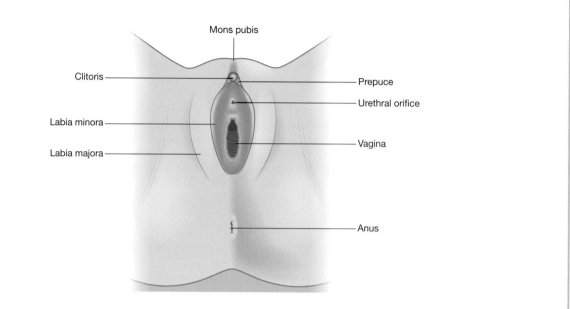

Anatomy and Physiology for Nurses at a Glance, First Edition. Ian Peate and Muralitharan Nair. © 2015 John Wiley & Sons, Ltd. Published 2015 by John Wiley & Sons, Ltd.
Companion website: www.ataglanceseries.com/nursing/anatomy

The external female genitalia are known collectively as the vulva. They include the mons pubis, the labia, the clitoris, the vaginal and urethral openings, and glands (see Figure 39.1). The external genitalia have three key functions:

1 Enabling sperm to enter the body.
2 Protecting the internal genital organs from infectious organisms.
3 The provision of sexual pleasure.

The mons veneris

The mons veneris is Latin for 'hill of Venus' (Venus was the Roman Goddess of love); it is the pad of elevated fatty tissue covering the pubic bone this is situated inferior (below) the abdomen and superior (above) to the labia. The amount of fat increases during puberty and after the menopause it decreases. The mons acts in such a way as to protect the pubic bone (the symphysis pubis is the name given to where two bones meet at the front of the pelvis) from the impact of sexual intercourse. During puberty the mons is covered with coarse pubic hair, after puberty this decreases.

Labia majora

These are the outer lips of the vulva and they are made of two symmetrical pads of fatty tissue that wrap around the vulva extending from the mons to the perineum. They provide protection for the urethral and vaginal openings. It is usual for these labia to be covered with pubic hair, they contain a number of sweat and oil glands, the scent (pheromones), from these glands may have a role to play in sexual arousal.

Labia minora

The inner lips of the vulva are known as the labia minora, composed of thin stretches of tissue within the labia majora, folding and protecting the vagina, urethra and the clitoris. They are thin, delicate folds of fat free hairless skin located between the labia majora. The labia minora contain a core of spongy tissue and within this there are many small blood vessels but no fat. The appearance of the labia minora varies from woman to woman, from tiny lips that are hidden between the labia majora to larger lips that can protrude. Internally the surface consists of thin skin and has a pink colour associated with mucous membranes. It contains a number of sensory nerve endings. Both the inner and outer labia are very sensitive to touch and pressure.

Clitoris

The clitoris is a small white aspect of oval tissue that is located at the top of the labia minora and the clitoral hood. The clitoris is a small body of spongy tissue and is highly sexually sensitive. Externally it is only the tip or glans of the clitoris that is visible, the organ itself is elongated and then branches into two forks, the crura, this then extends downwards along the edge of the vaginal opening toward the perineum. On average the clitoris is approximately 3 cm in length. The external tip of the clitoris or the clitoral glans is protected by the prepuce, (also called the clitoral hood), a covering of tissue that is analogous to the foreskin of the male penis. The clitoris can extend and the hood retracts to make the clitoral glans more accessible during sexual excitement, the clitoris is an erectile organ and is usually hidden by the labia when flaccid. The clitoris will, like the penis, enlarge upon tactile stimulation; it does not however lengthen significantly. It is highly sensitive and very important in the sexual arousal of a female. There are variations in size with some women and the clitoral glans may be very small in other women they may have a large clitoris and the hood may not completely cover it. The clitoris is suspended by a suspensory ligament.

The urethra

The external urethral orifice is located 2 to 3 cm posterior to the clitoris and immediately anterior to the vaginal orifice. The openings of the ducts of the paraurethral glands (also called Skene's glands) are located on each side of the vaginal orifice. These glands are said to be homologous to the male prostate gland. The urethra is not related to sex or reproduction, it is where urine is excreted when it passed from the urinary bladder.

Hymen

The hymen is pinkish; it is often shaped like a crescent, though there may be many other forms. It is a thin membrane found at the lower end of the vagina. In nearly all young women, there is a large gap in the membrane. In other words, it does not block off the vagina completely. This is important, because the hole in the hymen allows the menstrual blood to come through when the girl starts having periods. The hymen is the traditional symbol of virginity; as it is a very thin membrane, it can be torn by vigorous exercise, the insertion of a tampon, masturbation or the use of sex toys such as dildos.

Blood supply
Arterial supply of the female external genitalia

The rich arterial supply to the vulva comes from two external pudendal arteries as well as one internal pudendal artery located on either side. The internal pudendal artery supplies the skin, sex organs and the perineal muscles. The labial arteries are branches of the internal pudendal artery, and this is the same for the dorsal and deep arteries of the clitoris.

Venous drainage of the female external genitalia

The labial veins are offshoots of the internal pudendal veins and venae comitantes of the internal pudendal artery.

Lymph drainage

Within the vulva there are a number of very rich networks of lymphatic channels. The majority of lymph vessels pass to the superficial inguinal lymph nodes and deep inguinal nodes.

Nerve supply

The nerves that supply the vulva are branches of:

1 The ilioinguinal nerve.
2 The genital branch of the genitofemoral nerve.
3 The perineal branch of the femoral cutaneous nerve.
4 The perineal nerve.

40 The breast

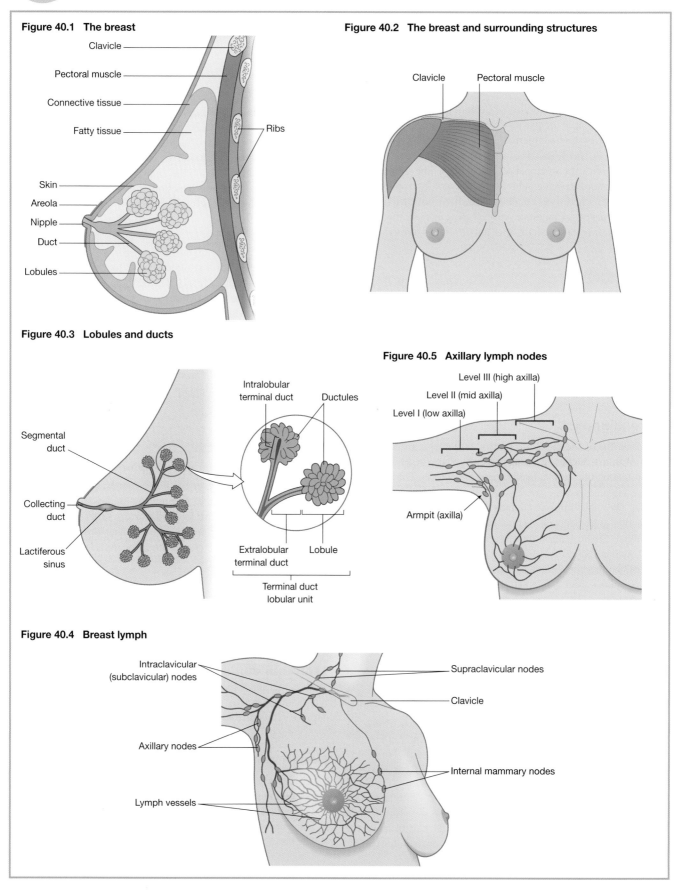

Figure 40.1   The breast

Clavicle
Pectoral muscle
Connective tissue
Fatty tissue
Ribs
Skin
Areola
Nipple
Duct
Lobules

Figure 40.2   The breast and surrounding structures

Clavicle   Pectoral muscle

Figure 40.3   Lobules and ducts

Segmental duct
Collecting duct
Lactiferous sinus

Intralobular terminal duct
Ductules
Extralobular terminal duct
Lobule
Terminal duct lobular unit

Figure 40.5   Axillary lymph nodes

Level III (high axilla)
Level II (mid axilla)
Level I (low axilla)
Armpit (axilla)

Figure 40.4   Breast lymph

Intraclavicular (subclavicular) nodes
Supraclavicular nodes
Clavicle
Axillary nodes
Internal mammary nodes
Lymph vessels

Anatomy and Physiology for Nurses at a Glance, First Edition. Ian Peate and Muralitharan Nair. © 2015 John Wiley & Sons, Ltd. Published 2015 by John Wiley & Sons, Ltd.
Companion website: www.ataglanceseries.com/nursing/anatomy

The breast is a part of the female external reproductive system. Women and men both have breasts, however women have more breast tissue than men.

The breast

Function

The key function of the breast is to produce, store and release milk to feed a baby. Milk is produced in lobules that are located throughout the breast after they have been stimulated by hormones produced in the woman's body after she has given birth. The milk is carried to the nipple by the ducts and from the nipple to the baby during breast-feeding.

Structure

The structure of the female breast is complex, within it there is fat and connective tissue, as well as lobes, lobules, ducts and lymph nodes (see Figure 40.1). The breast lies over a muscle of the chest known as the pectoral muscle. The female breast covers a large area; it extends from just below the collarbone (clavicle), to the armpit (axilla) and across to the breastbone (sternum) (see Figure 40.2). The breast is a mass of glandular, fatty and connective tissue.

Lobules and ducts

Each breast contains a number of lobules (sections) that branch out from the nipple, the lobules are the glands that produce milk. A lobule holds tiny, hollow alveoli linked by a network of thin ducts (see Figure 40.3). During breast-feeding, the ducts carry milk from the alveoli toward the breast areola (the dark area of skin in the centre of the breast). From the areola, the ducts join together into larger ducts that terminate at the nipple. The areola (pink or brown in colour) is the circular area around the nipple, this contains small sweat glands which secrete moisture, this acts as a lubricant during breast-feeding. The nipple is the area found at the centre of the areola where the milk emerges

Fat, ligaments and connective tissue

The spaces around the lobules and ducts are filled with fat, ligaments and connective tissue. The amount of fat in the breast determines their size; the fat gives shape to the breast. In all women the actual milk-producing structures are nearly the same. Cyclic changes in hormone levels have an impact on breast tissue. In younger women it is usual for them to have denser and less fatty breast tissue than older women who have gone through the menopause. Ligaments provide support to the breast. They run from the skin through the breast attaching themselves to muscles on the chest.

Nerve supply

There are a number of major nerves in the breast area, these include nerves in the chest and arm. There are also sensory nerves in the skin of the chest and axilla. Branches from the 4th, 5th and 6th thoracic nerves supply the breasts.

Arteries and capillaries

Arterial blood supply to the breast comes from the thoracic branches of the axillary arteries and the internal mammary and intercostal arteries. Venous drainage of the breast is primarily accomplished by the axillary vein. The subclavian, intercostal and internal thoracic veins also aid in returning blood to the heart.

Lymph nodes and lymph ducts

The lymphatic system is a network of lymph nodes and lymph ducts that help to fight infection (see Figure 40.4). Axillary lymph nodes are located above the clavicle, behind the sternum as well as in other parts of the body. Lymph circulates throughout body tissues picking up fats, bacteria and other unwanted materials and filtering them out through the lymphatic system. Breast lymph nodes include, supraclavicular nodes – above the clavical; infraclavicular (or subclavicular) nodes – below the clavicle; axillary nodes – in the axilla and internal mammary nodes – inside the chest around the sternum.

There are about 30–50 lymph nodes in the axilla. This number varies from woman to woman. The axillary lymph nodes are divided into three levels depending on how close they are to the pectoral muscle on the chest (see Figure 40.5):
• Level I (low axilla) – in the lower or bottom aspect of the axilla, along the outside border of the pectoral muscle.
• Level II (mid axilla) – in the middle part of the axilla, under the pectoral muscle.
• Level III (high axilla) – below and near the centre of the clavicle, above the breast area and along the inside border of the pectoral muscle.

Breast development

At different times during a woman's life breast tissue changes. Changes occur during puberty, during the menstrual cycle, during pregnancy and after menopause. Female breasts do not begin growing until puberty, at this time the breasts respond to hormonal changes, predominantly increases in oestrogen and progesterone and they begin to develop. During puberty, breast ducts and milk glands grow. The breast skin stretches as the breasts grow, creating a rounded appearance. Young women tend to have more glandular tissue than older women. Most of the glandular and ductal tissue in older women is replaced with fatty tissue and breasts become less dense. Ligaments lose their elasticity as the woman ages, causing the breasts to sag. Size and shape of women's breasts vary considerably. A woman's breasts are rarely the same size; one breast is often slightly larger or smaller, higher or lower or shaped differently than the other.

Hormones and the breast

The main female hormone is oestrogen, it affects female sexual characteristics, such as breast development, and it is necessary for reproduction. The ovaries make up most of the oestrogen in a woman's body; a small amount is made by the adrenal glands. Progesterone (the other female sex hormone) is made in the ovaries. Progesterone prepares the uterus for pregnancy and the breasts for producing milk for breast-feeding (lactation). Each month breast tissues are exposed to cycles of oestrogen and progesterone throughout a woman's childbearing years. In the first part of the menstrual cycle, oestrogen stimulates the growth of the milk ducts. Progesterone takes over in the second part stimulating the lobules. Post menopause, the monthly cycle ends. The adrenal glands however, continue to produce oestrogen and a woman keeps her sexual characteristics.

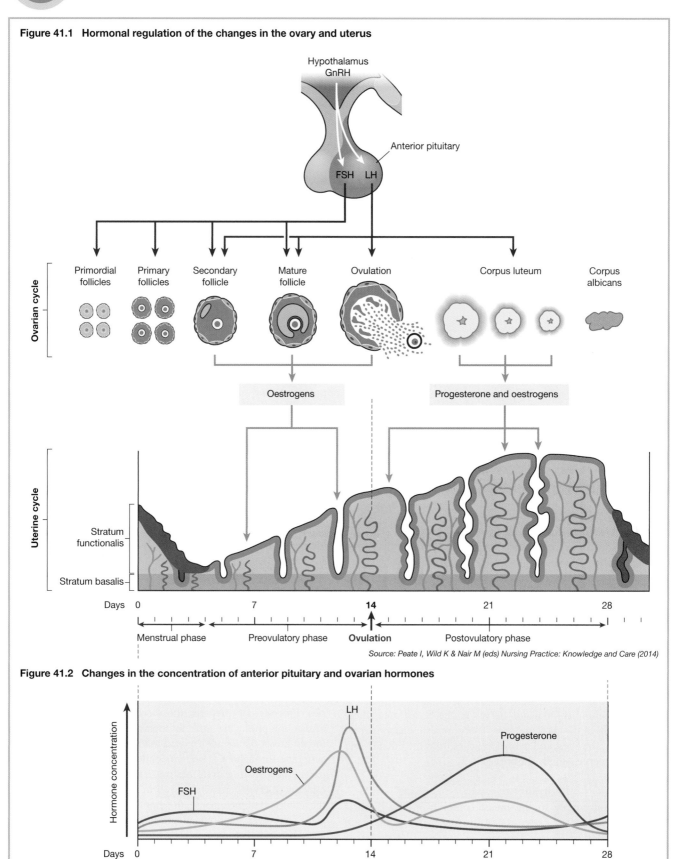

41 The menstrual cycle

Figure 41.1 Hormonal regulation of the changes in the ovary and uterus

Source: Peate I, Wild K & Nair M (eds) Nursing Practice: Knowledge and Care (2014)

Figure 41.2 Changes in the concentration of anterior pituitary and ovarian hormones

Source: Peate I, Wild K & Nair M (eds) Nursing Practice: Knowledge and Care (2014)

Anatomy and Physiology for Nurses at a Glance, First Edition. Ian Peate and Muralitharan Nair. © 2015 John Wiley & Sons, Ltd. Published 2015 by John Wiley & Sons, Ltd.
Companion website: www.ataglanceseries.com/nursing/anatomy

The reproductive cycle

The menstrual cycle is the series of changes that a woman's body goes through to prepare for a pregnancy. The key participants in the female reproductive cycle are the pituitary gland, the ovaries and the uterus and the activities of each are very closely coordinated.

The reproductive cycle encompasses a series of events that occur regularly every 26 to 30 days throughout the child-bearing period. Each month one of the ovaries releases a single egg: this is called ovulation. This occurs as a result of a complex set of interactions.

There are three sets of hormones that control the menstrual cycle:

1 Gonadotrophin-releasing hormones – luteinising hormone-releasing hormone (LHRH) and follicle-stimulating hormone-releasing hormone (FSHRH).

2 Gonadotrophins – luteinising hormone (LH) and follicle-stimulating hormone (FSH).

3 Ovarian hormones – oestrogen and progesterone.

Figure 41.1 provides an overview of the hormonal regulation of the changes in the ovary and uterus. Figure 41.2 describes the changes in the concentration of anterior pituitary and ovarian hormones.

The pituitary gland

The hypothalamus controls the actions of the pituitary gland; the menstrual cycle begins when the nerve cells in the hypothalamus trigger the secretion of the follicle stimulating hormone (FSH) and luteinising hormone (LH). The gonadotrophin hormone-releasing factors from the hypothalamus control the release of the pituitary hormones (the gonadotrophins) – FSH and LH. They are produced by the anterior pituitary gland and control the ovarian hormones oestrogen and progesterone.

The follicular phase

Also known as the proliferative phase, this is considered the first phase of the menstrual cycle that leads to ovulation: it is when the ovary prepares to release an egg. The cycle usually lasts for 28 days and the follicular phase is the first 14 days of the cycle. During the follicular phase there is a rise in FSH from the pituitary gland that stimulates the development of several follicles on the surface of the ovary, the follicles contain an egg. As the FSH level decreases, only one of the follicles continues to develop. This follicle also produces oestrogen. The endometrium prepares itself for the egg. In the early follicular phase, when menstrual flow has ended, the lining of the uterus is at its most thinest and levels of oestrogen and progesterone are at their lowest. Further on in the follicular phase, proliferation (or thickening) of the uterine lining happens.

The ovulatory phase

Ovulation is the key event of the menstrual cycle. During each cycle, only one egg/ovule is released from the dominant ovarian follicle as it responds to a surge in LH and can only be fertilised for up to 48 hours.

This phase of the cycle occurs when there is a surge in pituitary LH secretion and concludes with the extrusion of the mature ovum through the capsule of the ovary

The LH peaks mid-cycle, this then triggers the release of the ovum (this is ovulation), this usually happens 16 to 32 hours after the surge of LH begins. A couple of days later the levels of LH fall. The oestrogen level from the ovaries increases gradually towards ovulation and peaks during the LH surge, this is key to ovulation.

The levels of progesterone starts to rise towards follicle release, this prepares the endometrial lining of the uterus for implantation.

The luteal phase

During post-ovulation, known as the luteal phase or the premenstrual phase, the levels of LH and FSH decrease. The ruptured follicle closes (before doing this it releases the ovum) and forms a corpus luteum; the corpus luteum produces large amounts of progesterone. These large amounts of progesterone prevent oestrogen from stimulating another surge of LH from the pituitary gland. If the ovum is fertilised, the progesterone levels are maintained by the corpus luteum and the endometrium is maintained.

If the egg is fertilised by sperm and then implants in (or attaches to) the endometrium, a pregnancy begins. This pregnancy is dated from Day 1 of this menstrual cycle. If the fertilisation of the egg does not occur the corpus luteum starts to degenerate and progesterone and oestrogen levels begin to fall. The endometrial blood vessels constrict and the endometrial lining breaks down and is shed.

The menstrual cycle

The first day of the cycle is counted as the first day of the bleed – Day 1. The cycle runs from the first day of menstruation to the next first day; 28 days is the average cycle length, it is however normal to have a cycle that is shorter or longer. A teenager's cycles may be long (up to 45 days), becoming shorter over several years. Between 25 and 35 years, most women's cycles are regular and they generally last 21 to 35 days. At about 40 to 42, cycles tend to be the shortest and most regular. This is followed by 8 to 10 years of longer, less predictable cycles until menopause occurs.

Menstruation is largely an endometrial event and is prompted by the loss of progesterone provided by the corpus luteum that occurs in non-conception cycles. In the endometrium there are extraordinary structural changes that occur during menstruation, some of these changes are understood, however others are not.

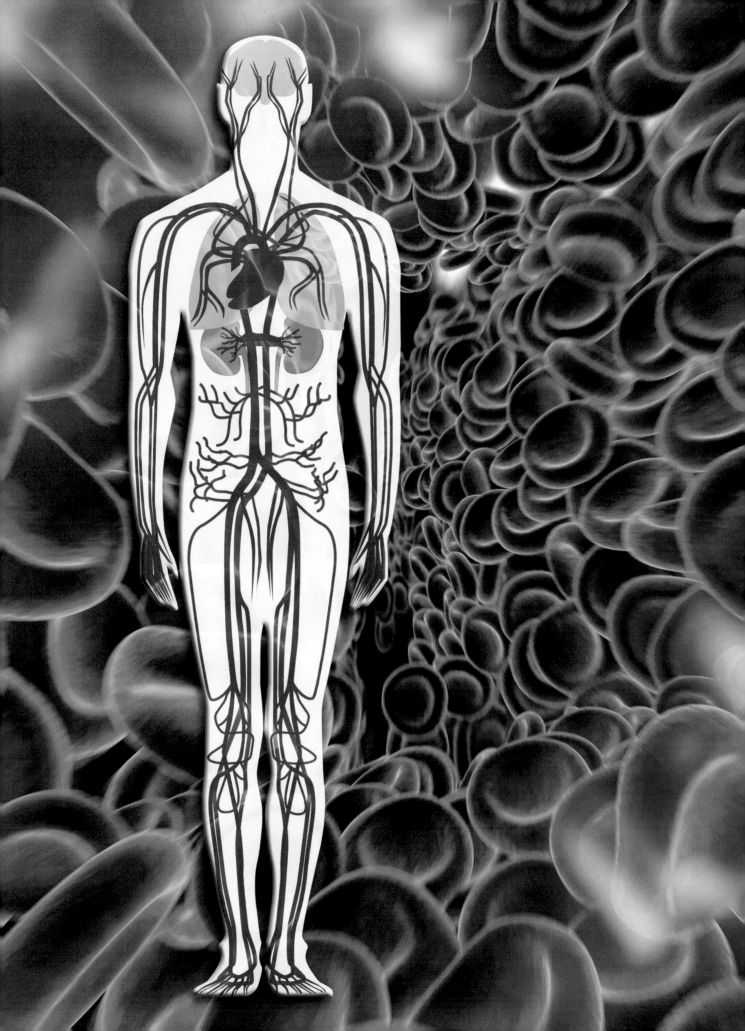

The endocrine system

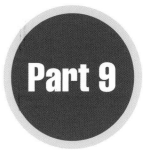

Part 9

Chapters

42 The endocrine system

Figure 42.1 The major endocrine glands

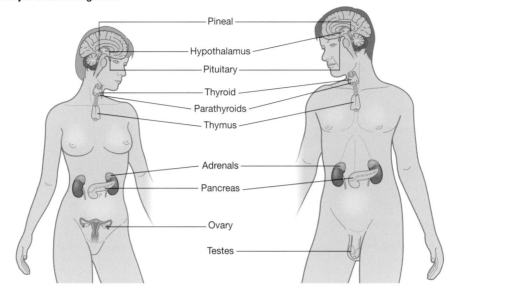

Pineal
Hypothalamus
Pituitary
Thyroid
Parathyroids
Thymus
Adrenals
Pancreas
Ovary
Testes

Figure 42.2 The pituitary gland and surrounding structures

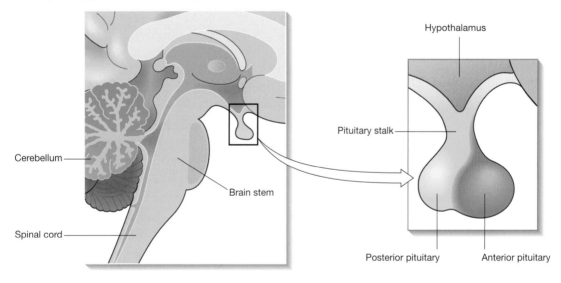

Cerebellum

Brain stem

Spinal cord

Hypothalamus

Pituitary stalk

Posterior pituitary   Anterior pituitary

Table 42.1 Hormones released by the hypothalamus and anterior pituitary gland

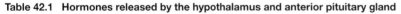

Hypothalamus	Anterior pituitary gland	Target organ or tissues	Action
Growth hormone releasing factor (GHRF)	Growth hormone (GH)	Various (particularly bone)	Stimulates the growth of body cell
Growth hormone release inhibiting factor (GHRIF)	Growth hormone (inhibits release)	Various	
Thyroid releasing hormone (TRH)	Thyroid stimulating hormone (TSH)	Thyroid gland	Stimulates thyroid hormone release
Corticotrophin releasing hormones (CRH)	Adrenocorticotropic hormone (ACTH)	Adrenal cortex	Stimulates the release of corticosteroid
Prolactin releasing hormone (PRH)	Prolactin	Breasts	Stimulates the production of milk
Prolactin inhibiting hormone	Prolactin (inhibits release)	Breasts	
Gonadotropin releasing hormone (GRH)	Follicle stimulating hormone Luteinising hormone	Gonads	Numerous reproductive functions

Anatomy and Physiology for Nurses at a Glance, First Edition. Ian Peate and Muralitharan Nair. © 2015 John Wiley & Sons, Ltd. Published 2015 by John Wiley & Sons, Ltd.
Companion website: www.ataglanceseries.com/nursing/anatomy

There are ten major endocrine glands (see Figure 42.1).

The endocrine glands

The endocrine system is not as closely linked as other systems, for example the circulatory system. Endocrine glands are groups of secretory cells that are surrounded by a large network of capillaries, this rich blood supply permits diffusion of hormones (see Table 42.1). In general, endocrine glands are ductless, vascular and most of them usually contain intracellular vacuoles or granules that store hormones. Exocrine glands however, for example the salivary glands, the mammary glands, sweat glands and those glands located within the gastrointestinal tract (for example, mucus glands), are usually much less vascular with a duct or lumen to a membrane surface.

The pituitary gland and the hypothalamus

The hypothalamus is an aspect of the brain that has a number of functions; it is one of the most important parts of the nervous system. The pituitary gland is approximately 1 cm in diameter (the size of a pea) and is cone shaped (Figure 42.2). It rests in the hypophyseal fossa, a depression in the sphenoid bone under the hypothalamus. The gland is connected to the hypothalamus by a slender stalk called the infundibulum. The pituitary gland and the hypothalamus act as a unit, controlling most of the other endocrine glands. Within the gland there are two distinct areas: the anterior lobe (adenohypophysis) composed of glandular epithelium and the posterior lobe (neurohypophysis) made of a down growth of nervous tissue from the brain. Arterial blood supply is from the internal carotid artery with venous drainage (containing hormones) leaving the gland via short veins that enter the venous sinuses between the layers in the dura mater. The activity of the adenohypophysis is controlled by the release of hormones from the hypothalamus. The neurohypophysis is controlled by nerve stimulation.

The pineal gland

The pineal gland secretes the hormone melatonin when sleeping, this influences circadian rhythm (this is roughly a 24 hour cycle in the physiological processes of humans), the pinealocytes synthesise melatonin directly into the cerebrospinal fluid, which then takes it into the blood. Secretion of the hormone is controlled by daylight with levels fluctuating throughout the day and seasons.

The anterior pituitary lobe

The anterior pituitary lobe (influenced by the hypothalamus) is supplied by arterial blood that has passed through the hypothalamus; blood is transported away from the gland via the pituitary portal system. The anterior pituitary lobe secretes a number of hormones. The anterior pituitary lobe is larger than the posterior lobe, and is made up of three parts; this partially surrounds the posterior lobe and infundibulum. This lobe is made up of glandular tissue producing and releasing hormones. There are no direct nerve connections with the anterior pituitary and the hypothalamus.

Control of the anterior pituitary occurs when releasing and inhibiting factors in the form of hormones are released by the hypothalamus.

Growth hormone (GH) stimulates the growth of bones, muscles and other organs by promoting protein synthesis. This hormone significantly affects the appearance of an individual as GH influences height.

Thyroid-stimulating hormone (TSH) causes the glandular cells of the thyroid to secrete thyroid hormone. If there is a hyper secretion of thyroid-stimulating hormone, the thyroid gland enlarges secreting excessive amounts of thyroid hormone.

Adrenocorticotropic hormone (ACTH) reacts with receptor sites located in the cortex of the adrenal gland stimulating the secretion of cortical hormones.

Gonadotropic hormones react with receptor sites in the gonads, regulating the development, growth and function of the testes or ovaries.

Prolactin hormone encourages the development of glandular tissue in the female breast during pregnancy and stimulates the production of milk after the birth of the child.

The posterior pituitary lobe

The posterior pituitary is primarily composed of nerve fibres (nerve bundle) that originate in hypothalamus; the supporting nerve cells are called pituicytes. The hypothalamic–hypophyseal tract links the posterior pituitary and the hypothalamus (this is the nerve bundle). The posterior pituitary releases two hormones, these hormones arrive directly from the hypothalamus:

1 oxytocin
2 antidiuretic hormone (ADH).

Oxytocin causes contraction of the smooth muscle in the wall of the uterus. It also stimulates the discharge of milk from the lactating breast; this is called the 'let down' response and occurs in response to suckling when milk is released. The role of this hormone in males and non-lactating females is unclear; however, oxytocin in men and women is thought to play a role in sexual arousal and orgasm.

The key role of ADH (vasopressin) is to reduce urinary output. ADH promotes the reabsorption of water by acting on the distal convoluted tubules and collecting ducts of the nephrons of the kidneys causing an increasing permeability to water. The result is that less water is lost as urine as reabsorption of water from the glomerular filtrate is increased. The amount of ADH that is secreted is controlled by the osmotic pressure of circulating blood to the osmoreceptors located in the hypothalamus. This mechanism conserves water for the body. Insufficient amounts of ADH cause excessive water loss in the urine. ADH secretion is stimulated by:

• increased plasma osmolality
• decreased extracellular volume
• pain and other stress conditions
• response to some drugs

When there is a high concentration of ADH, for example after excessive blood loss or severe dehydration, smooth muscle contracts and vasoconstriction in small arteries occurs. This results in the pressor effect where systemic blood pressure is elevated.

43 The thyroid and adrenal glands

Figure 43.1 The thyroid and parathyroid glands

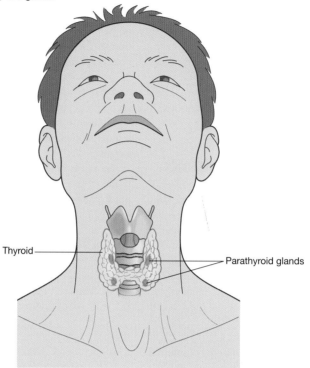

Thyroid —

— Parathyroid glands

Table 43.1 Some effects associated with an abnormal secretion of thyroid hormones

Increased secretion of T3 and T4 (hyperthyroidism)	Decreased secretion of T3 and T4 (hypothyroidism)
Increased basal metabolic rate	Decreased basal metabolic rate
Weight loss (despite good/increased appetite)	Weight gain (despite anorexia)
Tachycardia, palpitations, arrhythmia	Bradycardia
Excitability, nervousness, irritability	Tiredness, depression
Tremor	Numbness in the hands
Hair loss	Lifeless hair
Changes in menstruation patterns	Irregular menstrual periods
Goitre	Deep voice
Diarrhoea	Constipation
Exophthalmos	Feeling cold

Figure 43.2 Control of thyroid hormone production – negative feedback

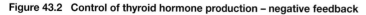

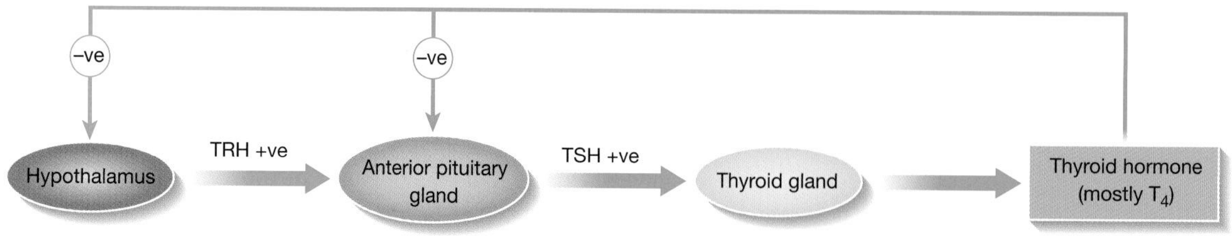

–ve   –ve

Hypothalamus → TRH +ve → Anterior pituitary gland → TSH +ve → Thyroid gland → Thyroid hormone (mostly T$_4$)

Source: Peate I & Nair M Fundamentals of Anatomy and Physiology for Student Nurses (2011)

The thyroid gland

The thyroid gland is located in the neck, anterior to the larynx and the trachea, situated at the level of the 5th, 6th and 7th cervical vertebrae and the 1st thoracic vertebra. This is a butterfly shaped gland (Figure 43.1) with two lobes comprised on either side of the thyroid cartilage and the upper incomplete cartilaginous rings of the trachea of a fibrous capsule weighing approximately 25 g. The gland is brownish red in colour. Lying in front of the trachea is the narrow isthmus joining the left and right lobes. Each lobe is cone shaped, measuring approximately 5 cm long and 3 cm wide. The upper aspects of the lobe are known as the upper poles and lower ends the lower poles. The lobes are compromised of hollow spherical shaped follicles surrounded by capillaries.

The blood supply to this gland is extensive (it is said to be a highly vascular gland). The arterial blood supply comes from the superior and inferior thyroid arteries. Venous return is by the thyroid veins draining into the internal jugular vein.

Principal innervation originates from the autonomic nervous system. Parasympathetic fibres come from the vagus nerves; sympathetic fibres are distributed from the superior, middle and inferior ganglia of the sympathetic trunk. These small nerves enter the gland accompanied by the blood vessels. Autonomic nervous regulation of the glandular secretion is not fully understood.

Lying against the posterior surfaces of each lobe are the parathyroid glands embedded in the thyroid tissues. The recurrent laryngeal nerve passes upwards and close to the lobes of the gland.

A single layer of epithelial cells comprise the follicles, these form a cavity containing thyroglobulin molecules that are attached to iodine molecules, the thyroid hormones are formed by these molecules. This gland releases two types of thyroid hormone, thyroxine (T_4) and triiodothyronine (T_3)

Iodine is essential for the synthesis of these hormones. Dietary iodine is concentrated by the thyroid gland, in the follicle cells it is changed into iodine. Thyroid stimulating hormone (TSH) simulates thyroid hormone production. The primary hormone released by the thyroid gland is T_4, this is converted into T_3 by the target cells. Thyroid hormones are required for normal growth and development. When there is deficiency of iodine, TSH is secreted in excess causing proliferation of thyroid gland cells accompanied by an enlargement of the gland. Table 43.1 outlines common effects associated with abnormal thyroid hormone secretion. Most of the cells in the body are affected by thyroid hormone, there is an increase in basal metabolic rate and production of heat.

The regulation of thyroid hormone secretion is via a negative feedback mechanism involving the amount of circulating hormone, hypothalamus and adenohypophysis (see Figure 43.2).

The parafollicular cells of the thyroid gland secrete calcitonin. Calcitonin combats the action of the parathyroid glands by reducing the levels of calcium in the blood. If blood calcium becomes too high, calcitonin is secreted until calcium ion levels decrease to normal.

Parathyroid glands

Four small masses of epithelial tissue embedded in the connective tissue capsule on the posterior surface of the thyroid glands are the parathyroid glands (Figure 43.1). They are responsible for the creation and secretion of parathyroid hormone, and are arranged in nests or cords around a dense capillary network. Parathyroid hormone is the most important regulator of blood calcium level. The key target cells are those in the bones and the kidneys, the hormone increases intestinal calcium absorption, stimulation of renal calcium absorption and the stimulation of osteoclast activity and as such the reabsorption of calcium from the bones. The hormone is secreted in response to low blood calcium levels and its effect is to increase those levels.

Hypoparathyroidism, or inadequate secretion of parathyroid hormone, leads to increased nerve excitability. The low blood calcium levels trigger spontaneous and continuous nerve impulses, which then stimulate muscle contraction. Calcium is also required for the creation of clotting factors in the blood which is monitored by cells in the gland. When there is a reduction in blood calcium levels this leads to an increase in the formation and secretion of parathyroid hormone.

The adrenal glands

The adrenal glands are located one each near the upper portion of each kidney. Each gland has an outer cortex and an inner medulla. The cortex and medulla, like the anterior and posterior lobes of the pituitary, secrete different hormones. The adrenal cortex is essential to life; the medulla may be removed with no life-threatening effects.

The hypothalamus influences both aspects of the adrenal gland but uses different mechanisms. The adrenal cortex is regulated by negative feedback involving the hypothalamus and adrenocorticotropic hormone; the medulla is regulated by nerve impulses from the hypothalamus.

Hormones of the adrenal cortex

The adrenal cortex consists of three different regions; each region produces a different group or type of hormone. All the cortical hormones are steroid.

The outermost region of the adrenal cortex secretes mineralacorticoids, aldosterone is the chief mineralocorticoid, conserving sodium ions and water in the body. The middle region of the adrenal cortex secretes glucocorticoids. The key glucocorticoid is cortisol, increasing levels of blood glucose.

The third group of steroids is the gonadocorticoids (sex hormones), secreted by the innermost region. Male hormones – androgens, and female hormones – oestrogens, are secreted in minimal amounts in both sexes by the adrenal cortex, their effect is often masked by hormones from the testes and ovaries. In females, the masculinisation effect of androgen secretion can become evident after menopause as levels of oestrogen from the ovaries decrease.

Hormones of the adrenal medulla

The adrenal medulla secretes two hormones, epinephrine and norepinephrine, in response to stimulation by sympathetic nerves, predominantly during stressful situations. A lack of hormones from the adrenal medulla will have no significant effects. Hypersecretion causes prolonged or continual sympathetic responses.

44 The pancreas and gonads

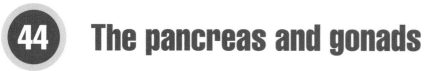

Figure 44.1   The pancreas

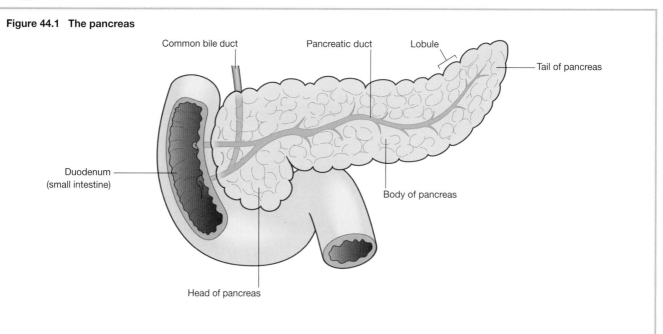

Common bile duct   Pancreatic duct   Lobule

Tail of pancreas

Duodenum
(small intestine)

Body of pancreas

Head of pancreas

Figure 44.2   Insulin and glucagon effects on blood glucose

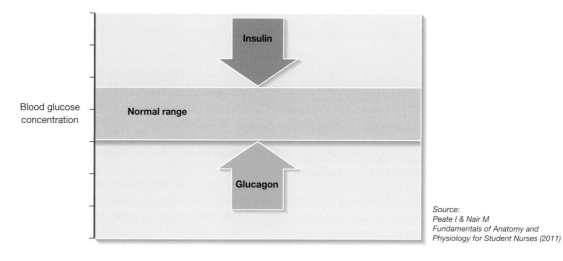

Blood glucose
concentration

Insulin

Normal range

Glucagon

Source:
Peate I & Nair M
Fundamentals of Anatomy and
Physiology for Student Nurses (2011)

Table 44.1   Other endocrine glands

Organ	Description
Thymus gland	Thymosin, a hormone produced by the thymus gland, has an important role in the development of the immune system
Stomach	The lining of the stomach, the gastric mucosa, produces gastrin, when food is present in the stomach. This stimulates the production of hydrochloric acid and the enzyme pepsin, used in the digestion of food
Small intestine	The mucosa of the small intestine secretes secretin and cholecystokinin when secreted promotes the pancreas to produce a fluid that neutralises the stomach acid. Cholecystokinin stimulates contraction of the gallbladder, releasing bile and stimulates the pancreas to secrete digestive enzyme
Heart	The heart also acts as an endocrine organ as well as pumping blood. Special cells in the wall of the atria produce atrial natriuretic hormone, or atriopeptin
Placenta	The placenta develops as a source of nourishment and gas exchange for the developing foetus. It also serves as a temporary endocrine gland. One hormone it secretes is human chorionic gonadotropin which signals the woman's ovaries to secrete hormones to maintain the uterine lining so that it does not degenerate and slough off in menstruation

Anatomy and Physiology for Nurses at a Glance, First Edition. Ian Peate and Muralitharan Nair. © 2015 John Wiley & Sons, Ltd. Published 2015 by John Wiley & Sons, Ltd.
Companion website: www.ataglanceseries.com/nursing/anatomy

The pancreas

The pancreas is located in the epigastric and left hypochondriac regions of the abdomen, the head of the pancreas lies close to the first part of the small intestine – the duodenum and the body behind the stomach, the tail extends out towards the spleen. It is about 12 to 15 cm in length and weighs approximately 60 g, the pancreas is a pale grey elongated gland (Figure 44.1).

Blood supply to the pancreas comes from the splenic and mesenteric arteries. The splenic and mesenteric arteries drain the pancreas where this drainage joins and forms the portal vein. The pancreas is innervated by the parasympathetic and sympathetic nervous systems. The secretion of insulin and glucagon is stimulated by the nervous system.

This gland has both endocrine and exocrine functions. Most of the tissue within the pancreas is made up of exocrine tissue and the associated ducts.

The exocrine pancreas

The exocrine aspect of the gland is made up of a number of lobules composed of acini secreting digestive enzymes that are carried through a duct to the duodenum. The function of the exocrine element is to produce pancreatic juice that is rich in enzymes whose responsibility is to digest carbohydrates, protein and fats.

The endocrine pancreas

The endocrine portion scattered throughout the exocrine tissue consists of the pancreatic islets (the islets of Langerhans). The islets are the endocrine cells of the pancreas, which secrete insulin and glucagon, the islets have no ducts; the hormones are diffused directly into the blood. The islets have three key cell types producing a different hormone:

1 Alpha cells secreting glucagon.
2 Beta cells secreting insulin – these are the most abundant of the three cell types.
3 Delta cells secrete somatostatin.

All three cell types are specifically placed within the islets' beta cells and are located in the central aspect of the islet surrounded by the alpha and delta cells. As the islets are highly vascularised this enables the transportation of the hormones into the blood to occur at speed.

Insulin

This hormone is responsible for a number of things (including its effect on protein and mineral and lipid metabolism); one of the most well known responsibilities is its ability to reduce blood glucose levels. Insulin facilitates the movement of glucose into muscle, adipose and other tissues (the brain and the liver do not require insulin for the uptake of glucose). Insulin stimulates the liver to store glucose as glycogen.

Insulin synthesis is in response (principally) to a rise in blood glucose levels and increases in blood, amino acids and fatty acids also have a stimulating effect. When blood glucose levels drop there is a matching drop in insulin production and secretion, glycogen synthesis in the liver is reduced and enzymes responsible for the breakdown of glycogen are activated.

Glucagon

This hormone is also responsible for the maintenance of normal blood glucose. Glucagon has the opposite effects on blood glucose to insulin (see Figure 44.2). Glucagon increases blood glucose levels by simulating the conversion of glycogen to glucose in the liver and skeletal muscles. Low blood sugar levels, exercise and decreased somatostatin and insulin stimulate the secretion of glucagon.

Somatostatin

This inhibits the release of insulin and glycogen; when this hormone is released it has effects locally. The exact way this hormone functions is unknown.

The gonads

The gonads are the primary reproductive organs: the testes in the male and the ovaries in the female. These organs are responsible for producing the sperm and ova and also secrete hormones and as such are considered endocrine glands.

The ovaries

Chapters 38 and 39 discuss the functions of the female reproductive system in detail.

The ovaries produce two groups of female sex hormones which are the oestrogens and progesterone. These are steroid hormones and contribute to the development and function of the female reproductive organs and sex characteristics. At the onset of puberty, oestrogens promote breast development, fat distribution and maturation of reproductive organs such as the uterus and vagina.

Progesterone causes the uterine lining to thicken in preparation for pregnancy. Progesterone and oestrogens are responsible for the changes occurring in the uterus during the female menstrual cycle.

The testes

Chapter 35 discusses the functions of the male reproductive system in detail.

Male sex hormones are called androgens. The main androgen is testosterone, secreted by the testes; the adrenal cortex also produces a small amount. Testosterone production starts during foetal development, continuing for a short time after birth, almost ceases during childhood and then at puberty resumes. This hormone is responsible for the growth and development of the male reproductive structures, increased skeletal and muscular growth, enlargement of the larynx accompanied by voice changes, growth and distribution of body hair and increased male sexual drive.

The secretion of testosterone is regulated by a negative feedback system involving the release of hormones from the hypothalamus and gonadotropins from the anterior pituitary.

Other endocrine glands

In addition to the major endocrine glands discussed in this chapter, other organs have some hormonal activity as part of their function. These include the thymus, stomach, small intestines, heart and placenta (see Table 44.1).

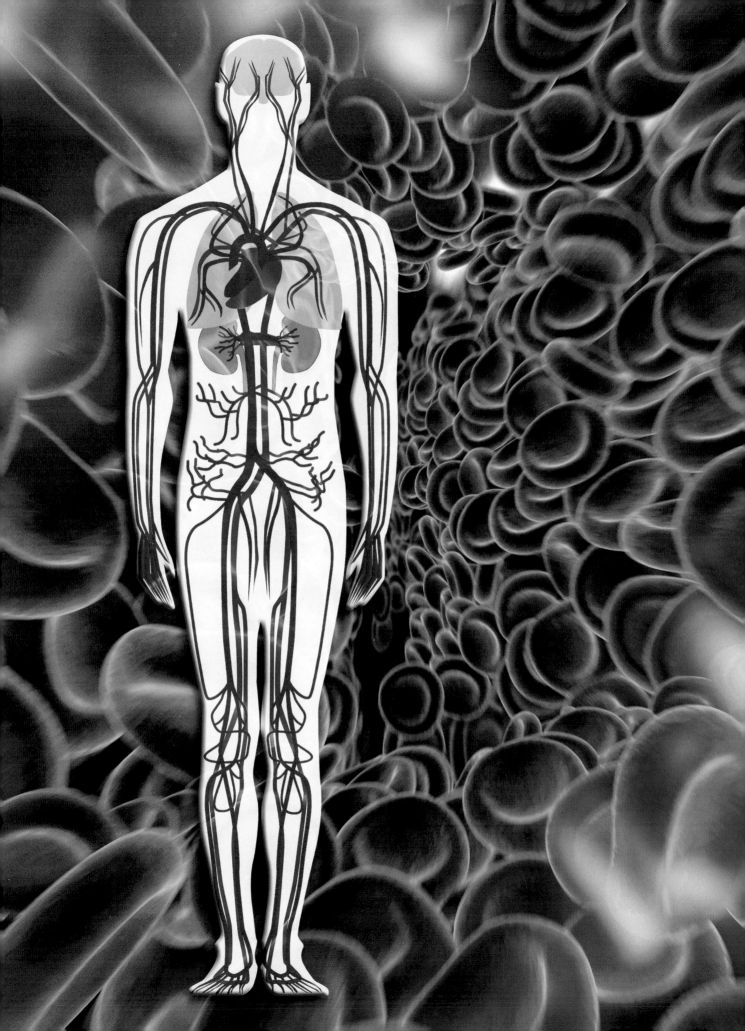

The musculoskeletal system

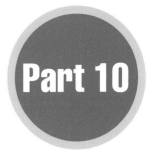

Part 10

Chapters

45 Bone structure

Figure 45.1 Bone remodelling

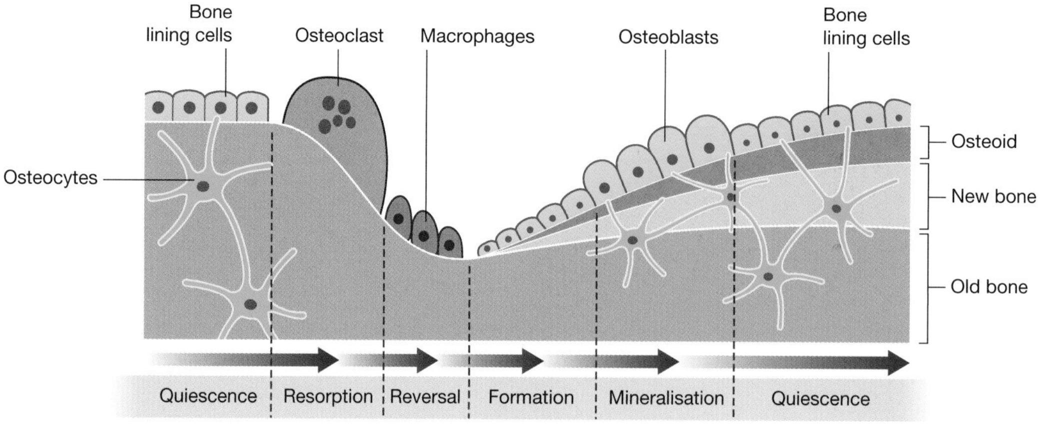

Bone lining cells · Osteoclast · Macrophages · Osteoblasts · Bone lining cells

Osteocytes

Osteoid
New bone
Old bone

Quiescence · Resorption · Reversal · Formation · Mineralisation · Quiescence

Source: Peate I, Wild K & Nair M (eds) Nursing Practice: Knowledge and Care (2014)

Figure 45.2 Bone growth

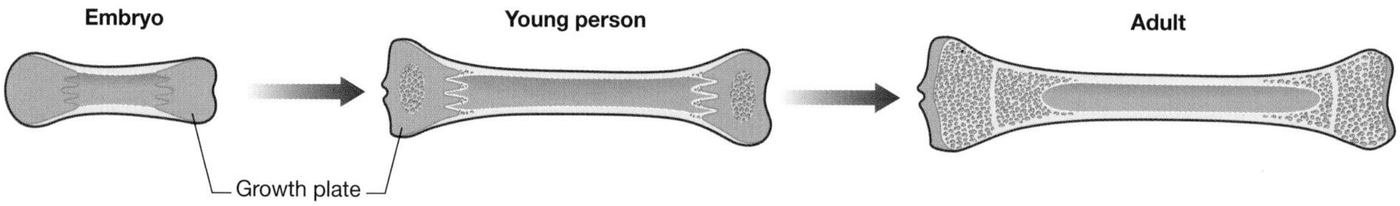

Embryo · **Young person** · **Adult**

Growth plate

Figure 45.3 Osteon, haversian canal

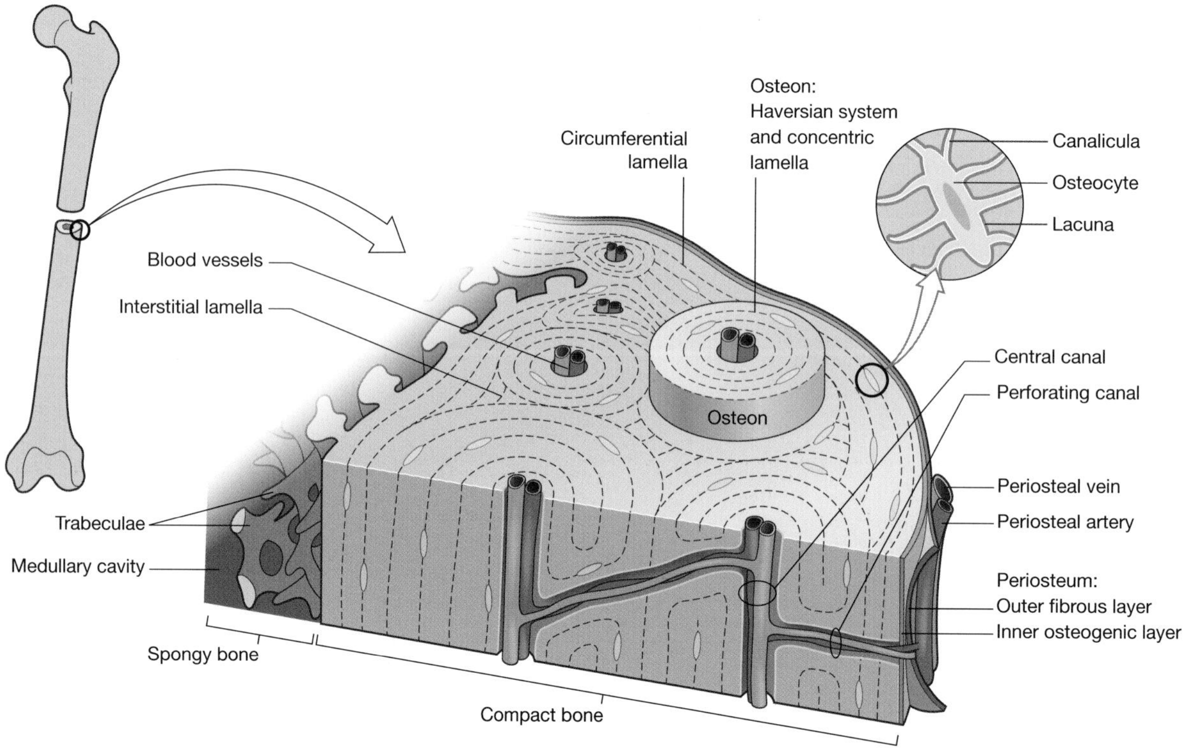

Circumferential lamella

Osteon: Haversian system and concentric lamella

Canalicula
Osteocyte
Lacuna

Blood vessels
Interstitial lamella

Osteon

Central canal
Perforating canal
Periosteal vein
Periosteal artery
Periosteum: Outer fibrous layer
Inner osteogenic layer

Trabeculae
Medullary cavity
Spongy bone

Compact bone

Source: Peate I, Wild K & Nair M (eds) Nursing Practice: Knowledge and Care (2014)

Anatomy and Physiology for Nurses at a Glance, First Edition. Ian Peate and Muralitharan Nair. © 2015 John Wiley & Sons, Ltd. Published 2015 by John Wiley & Sons, Ltd.
Companion website: www.ataglanceseries.com/nursing/anatomy

Bone is living material, made up of minerals, consisting of living tissue and non-living substances. Bone is a dynamic tissue that continues to be built, broken down and rebuilt in a process called bone remodelling.

Bone structure can be compared to reinforced concrete used to make a building or a bridge. When the building or bridge is first assembled, an initial frame is put in place containing long steel rods. Cement is then poured around the rods. The rods and the cement form a close-fitting union, creating a structure that is strong and resilient enough to survive a rocking motion whilst also maintaining strength. If the steel rods were not present, then the cement would be brittle and liable to fracture even when only minor movements are made. Without the cement the steel rods would have insufficient support, they would bend.

The same organisation is true of bone. The steel rods are the collagen rods in bone. The cement surrounding and supporting the rods are formed by minerals (calcium and phosphorous) from the blood that crystallise and surround the rods. Minerals provide the bones with strength and collagen rods flexibility.

Bone remodelling and modelling

The skeleton changes as we age, throughout childhood bone formation and growth occur with a gradual loss of bone density beginning in early adulthood and increasing significantly in older adults. During the process of ossification calcium is used to create bone as the child grows and matures. Gradually bone becomes hard and strong.

The density of bone is controlled by a group of cells including osteoclasts, these multi nucleated cells resorb bone. Osteoblasts refill the cavities created by osteoclasts.

Bone resorbtion and formation is known as remodelling. Bone modelling occurs when there is an increase in bone mass. Bone modelling promotes the growth of bones and is important for maintaining bone strength. Remodelling also plays an important part in bone growth by improving the growing structure (see Figure 45.1).

People over 30 years experience a gradual loss in bone mass as there is a decrease in the activity in osteoblasts compared with osteoclasts. A number of factors play a part in the decrease in bone mass; for example, the use of glucocorticoids enhances the activity of the osteoclasts, reducing bone formation. Loss of bone mass reduces strength and increases risk of fracture.

In the foetus, most of the skeleton is made up of cartilage, a tough, flexible connective tissue with no minerals or salts. As the foetus grows, osteoblasts and osteoclasts slowly replace cartilage cells, and ossification begins (see Figure 45.2).

Ossification

Ossification is the formation of bone by the activity of osteoblasts and osteoclasts and the addition of minerals and salts. Calcium compounds must be present for ossification to occur. Osteoblasts do not make these minerals, but take them from the blood and deposit them in bone. At birth, many of the bones have been at least partly ossified.

Within the bone are blood vessels, nerves, collagen and living cells including:
• osteoclasts
• osteoblasts

Osteoclasts

Bone tissue is continually broken down and resorbed by multi nuclear cells called osteoclasts, derived from monocytes which originate within bone marrow. Osteoclasts have an important role to play in liberating minerals and other molecules stored within the bone matrix.

Bone tissue serves as an important source of essential minerals including calcium and phosphate and other biological molecules such as growth factors. When calcium is released from the bone this plays a role in maintaining homeostasis.

Osteoclasts are regulated by different signalling pathways and molecules. Increased osteoclast activity leads to increased resorption of bone.

Osteoblasts

Osteoblasts are the cells responsible for building new bone tissue. These are derived from cells thought to be associated with blood vessels. When activation occurs they begin the production of the organic components of bone – osteoid this is predominantly made of collagen. Minerals begin to crystallise around the collagen scaffold forming the major inorganic constituent of bone which contains calcium phosphate.

As osteoblasts form, new bone tissue may become imbedded within the matrix differentiating into osteocytes.

The structures and processes occurring within bone allow it to serve concurrently as a calcium reservoir whilst also providing structural support for the vital organs and movement.

The skeleton

The skeleton provides the body with shape and physical support for the systems contained within. The skeleton forms part of the musculoskeletal system enabling us to move.

The interior of bone is composed of bone marrow, surrounded by:
• Cortical bone (the hard outer shell of bone).
• Trabecular bone (the spongy looking centre).

The amount of cortical of trabecular tissue is dependent upon the function of the bone. The osteon is the basic unit of structure of compact bone, comprising a Haversian canal and its concentrically arranged lamellae (see Figure 45.3).

Osteocytes are distributed within the lamellae, forming a network that maintains the viability and structural integrity of bone.

The Haversian canal is located at the centre of the osteons, containing blood vessels and nerves; blood vessels facilitate the exchange between osteocytes and blood. The vascular network provides structural support, nutrition and a waste removal system within this space.

Trabecular bone is present in the interior of some bones and resists compression; within the structure there are osteocytes, playing an important part in sensing local changes in strain.

In the interior of bones is the bone marrow. Bone marrow is a site for haematopoiesis, the process by which the cellular components of blood are formed.

46 Bone types

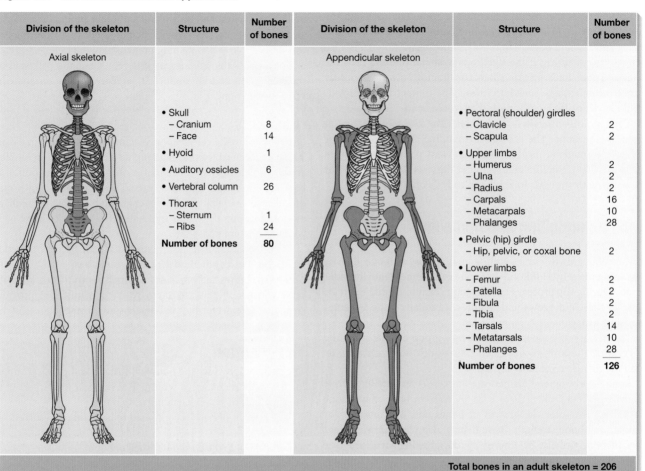

Figure 46.1 The skeleton: axial and appendicular

Division of the skeleton	Structure	Number of bones	Division of the skeleton	Structure	Number of bones
Axial skeleton			Appendicular skeleton		
	• Skull			• Pectoral (shoulder) girdles	
	– Cranium	8		– Clavicle	2
	– Face	14		– Scapula	2
	• Hyoid	1		• Upper limbs	
	• Auditory ossicles	6		– Humerus	2
	• Vertebral column	26		– Ulna	2
	• Thorax			– Radius	2
	– Sternum	1		– Carpals	16
	– Ribs	24		– Metacarpals	10
	Number of bones	**80**		– Phalanges	28
				• Pelvic (hip) girdle	
				– Hip, pelvic, or coxal bone	2
				• Lower limbs	
				– Femur	2
				– Patella	2
				– Fibula	2
				– Tibia	2
				– Tarsals	14
				– Metatarsals	10
				– Phalanges	28
				Number of bones	**126**

Total bones in an adult skeleton = 206

Source: Peate I, Wild K & Nair M (eds) Nursing Practice: Knowledge and Care (2014)

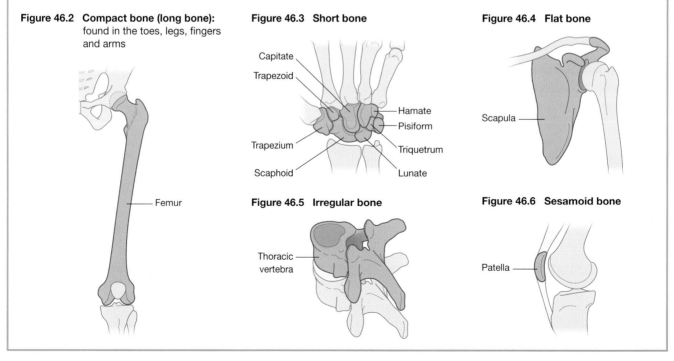

Figure 46.2 Compact bone (long bone): found in the toes, legs, fingers and arms

Femur

Figure 46.3 Short bone

Capitate
Trapezoid
Hamate
Pisiform
Trapezium
Triquetrum
Scaphoid
Lunate

Figure 46.4 Flat bone

Scapula

Figure 46.5 Irregular bone

Thoracic vertebra

Figure 46.6 Sesamoid bone

Patella

Anatomy and Physiology for Nurses at a Glance, First Edition. Ian Peate and Muralitharan Nair. © 2015 John Wiley & Sons, Ltd. Published 2015 by John Wiley & Sons, Ltd.
Companion website: www.ataglanceseries.com/nursing/anatomy

The human skeleton contains around 300 bones at birth, and by the time the person reaches adulthood this number has diminished to 206. As we age smaller bones join together to make bigger bones – they fuse. The bones give the body its shape. The main job of the skeleton is to provide support for the body. Without the skeleton the body would collapse into a pile. The skeleton is strong but light. See Figure 46.1 – the skeleton.

The skeleton also helps to protect the internal organs as well as the fragile body tissues. The skeleton protects the brain, eyes, heart, lungs and spinal cord. The cranium (the skull) offers protection to the brain and eyes, whilst the ribs protect the heart and lungs and the vertebrae the (spine, backbones) protect the spinal cord. Bones provide the structure for muscles to attach so that we are able to move. Tendons are tough inelastic bands that hold and attach muscle to bone. Red bone marrow makes blood cells and yellow marrow stores fat.

The study of bones is known as osteology.

Skeleton divisions

The bones are a major component of the skeletal system and are divided into two groups; these are the axial skeletal bones and appendicular skeletal bones. In an adult human skeleton there are 206 bones, 80 of which are from the axial skeleton and 126 from the appendicular skeleton.

The axial skeleton

The axial skeleton comprises the skull — includes bones of the cranium, face and ears (auditory ossicles). Hyoid – U-shaped bone or complex of bones located in the neck between the chin and larynx. Vertebral column – includes spinal vertebrae. Thoracic cage – includes ribs and sternum (breast bone).

The appendicular skeleton

The appendicular skeleton is comprised of body limbs and structures that attach limbs to the axial skeleton. Bones of the upper and lower limbs, pectoral girdles and pelvic girdle are elements of this aspect of the skeleton. Although the primary function of the appendicular skeleton is for bodily movement, it also provides protection for organs of the digestive system, excretory system, and reproductive system. The appendicular skeleton includes the pectoral girdle – includes shoulder bones (clavicle and scapula). Upper limbs – includes bones of the arms and hands. Pelvic girdle – includes hip bones. Lower limbs – includes bones of the legs and feet.

Bone types

Bone types can be classified according to the shape and size of the bone. The shapes of bones reflect their functions. It is useful when describing specific bones to begin by stating the type of bone in relation to its shape; for example, the scapula is a large, flat, triangular bone. In terms of bone shape there are five main types of bone:

1 long bones
2 short bones
3 flat bones
4 irregular bones
5 sesamoid bones.

Bone tissue is classified as either compact bone or spongy bone and depends on how the bone matrix and cells are organised. Compact bone forms the outer layer of all bones and most of the structure of long bones (see Figure 46.2); it provides few spaces and offers protection and support to the bones around which it is the outer layer as well as helping the long bones to bear the weight of the stress placed on them by body weight. Spongy bone (also called cancelleous bone) has no osteons, instead spongy bone consists of an irregular lattice of thin columns of trabeculae. Spaces between the trabeculae of some spongy bones are filled with red bone marrow.

Long bones

These bones are often curved to assist with strength; they are longer and wider than other bones and consist of a shaft and a variable number of extremities (endings). The femur, tibia, fibula, humerus, ulna and radius are examples of long bones (see Figure 46.2).

Short bones

Can be described as cube shaped and are approximately the same size length and width. Their primary function is to provide support and stability with little movement. Examples of short bones are the carpals and tarsals – the wrist and foot bones. These bones consist of only a thin layer of compact, hard bone with cancellous bone on the inside with relatively large amounts of bone marrow. See Figure 46.3.

Flat bones

Flat bones are strong, flat plates of bone whose key function is to provide protection to the body's vital organs as well as being a base for muscular attachment. A prime example of a flat bone is the scapula (shoulder blade). The sternum (breast bone), cranium (skull), os coxae (hip bone) pelvis and ribs are also classed as flat bones. The anterior and posterior surfaces are formed of compact bone with the intention of providing strength for protection; the centre consists of cancellous (spongy) bone with varying amounts of bone marrow. The greatest number of red blood cells are formed in flat bones in adults. See Figure 46.4.

Irregular bones

These bones do not fall into any other category, because of their non-uniform shape. Examples of these are the vertebrae, sacrum and mandible (lower jaw). They consist chiefly of cancellous bone, with a thin outer layer of compact bone. See Figure 46.5.

Sesamoid bones

These types of bones are mostly short or irregular bones, imbedded in a tendon. The patella (knee cap) is the most obvious example of this and sits within the patella or quadriceps tendon. Other types of sesamoid bones are the pisiform (smallest of the carpals) and the two small bones at the base of the first metatarsal. Sesamoid bones are usually present in a tendon where it passes over a joint; this provides protection for the tendon. See Figure 46.6.

Joints

Figure 47.1 Joint types

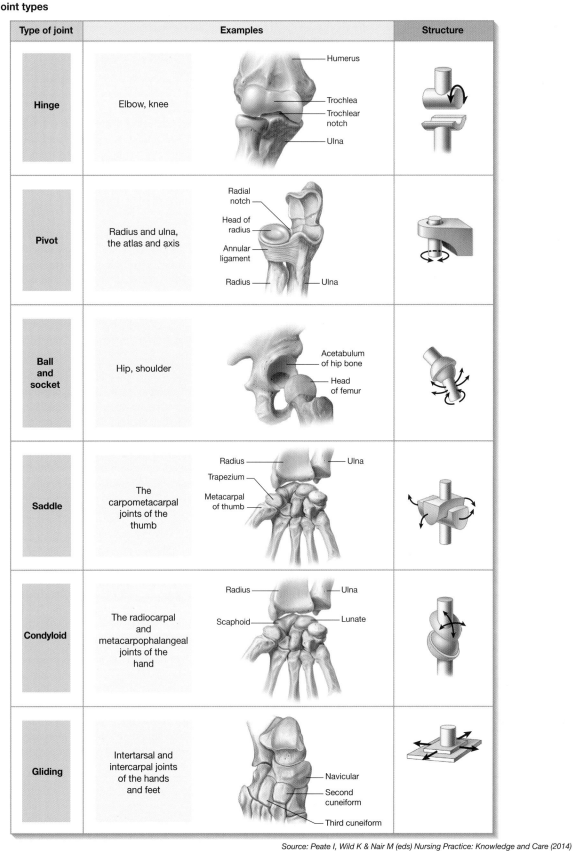

Source: Peate I, Wild K & Nair M (eds) Nursing Practice: Knowledge and Care (2014)

Joints are the place where two bones meet. All bones in the body (apart from the hyoid bone in the neck) form a joint with another bone. Joints hold the bones together permitting the rigid skeleton to move. Sometimes joints are also called articulations.

Movements

The skeleton allows movement. The bones act as levers providing the transmission of muscular forces, a number of bones can (through leverage, contracting and pulling) change the extent and direction of the forces that are generated by skeletal muscles, through the work of the tendons and the ligaments. These movements can be very intricate movements such as the ability to write, the ability to thread a needle (the coordination of fine movement) to gross movement such as the ability to move body position. The skeleton with the interaction of muscles enables breathing to occur. Movement becomes possible through articulation.

A tendon is a fibrous connective tissue attaching muscle to bone. Tendons can also attach muscles to structures such as the eyeball. A tendon helps to move the bone or structure. A ligament is a fibrous connective tissue attaching bone to bone, and generally serves to hold structures together, keeping them stable.

There are a number of different types of movement available at different joints, the shoulder joint, for example, moves in many more ways than the knee. These are the main types of movement:

• **Flexion:** Reducing the angle at the joint, bending the knee or elbow is flexion.
• **Extension:** Increasing the angle at the joint, for example, straightening the knee or elbow is extension.
• **Adduction:** Moving the body part towards the centre of the body, for example bringing one leg in towards the other is adduction.
• **Abduction:** Moving the body part away from the centre of the body, taking one leg away from the other is abduction.
• **Rotation:** Turning or twisting a body part, either clockwise (external or lateral) or anti-clockwise (internal or medial), for example, turning the leg to point the toes outwards.

Fibrous joints

These joints are also called synarthrodial joints. These joints are held together by only a ligament. A ligament is a dense irregular tissue that is made up of rich collagen fibres. There is no synovial cavity in this type of joint. Some examples of synarthrodial joints are where the teeth are held to their bony sockets, other examples include both the radioulnar and tibiofibular joints.

Cartilaginous joints

Cartilaginous joints are also known as synchondroses (the singular is synarthrosis) and symphyses (singular symphysis). They occur where the connection between the articulating bones are made up of cartilage with no synovial cavity, for example, the joints occurring between vertebrae in the spine.

The synchondroses are temporary joints and are only present in children up until the end of puberty, at this stage the hyaline cartilage is converted into bone, for example, the epiphyseal plates of long bones. Symphysis joints are permanent cartilagenous joints that have an intervening pad of fibrocartilage; for example, the symphysis pubis.

Synovial joints

Synovial joints, also called diarthrosis joints. are by far the most common classification of joint within the human body. These joints are extremely moveable with a synovial cavity and all have an articular capsule that encloses the whole joint, a synovial membrane (this is the inner layer of the capsule) which produces synovial fluid (a lubricating solution) and cartilage known as hyaline cartilage which pads the ends of the articulating bones.

Synovial fluid is a thin film that is usually viscous, clear or yellowish. The synovial fluid helps in preventing friction by providing the joint with lubrication, supplying nutrients and removing waste products. If the joint becomes immobile for a period of time then the fluid becomes gel like and when the joint begins to move again it returns to its usual viscous consistency.

Freely movable (synovial) joints

There are six types of freely moveable, or synovial joints (see Figure 47.1).

There are some joints, such as those in the skull, that are fixed and do not allow any movement to occur. The bones in the skull, for example, are held together with fibrous tissue, as are the joints in the pelvis.

The majority of joints are synovial joints which allow for much more movement than the cartilaginous joints. Synovial joints are mainly located in the limbs where mobility is essential. Ligaments help provide their stability and the muscles contract in order to produce movement.

Hinge

A convex portion of one bone fits into a concave portion of another bone. The movement reflects the hinge and bracket movement of a household hinge and bracket; movement is limited to flexion and extension. The joint produces an open and closing motion. These joints are uniaxial.

Pivot

A rounded part of one bone fits into the groove of another bone. These joints will only permit movement of one bone around another and are classified as uniaxial movement.

Ball and socket

The spherical end of one bone fits into a concave socket of another bone, hence the name ball and socket. Movement happens through flexion, extension and adduction. This is a triaxial joint.

Saddle

Similar to condyloid joints, but these joints permit greater movement. Allows flexion, extension and adduction. The joint is classed as triaxial.

Condyloid

Where an oval surface of one bone fits into a concavity of another bone and where condyloid joints are found. Permits flexion, extension and adduction. This kind of joint is a biaxial joint.

Gliding

These joints have a flat or slightly curved surface enabling gliding movements. The joints are bound by ligaments and movement in all directions is restricted. The joint moves back and forth and from side to side.

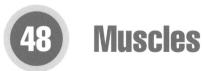

Muscles

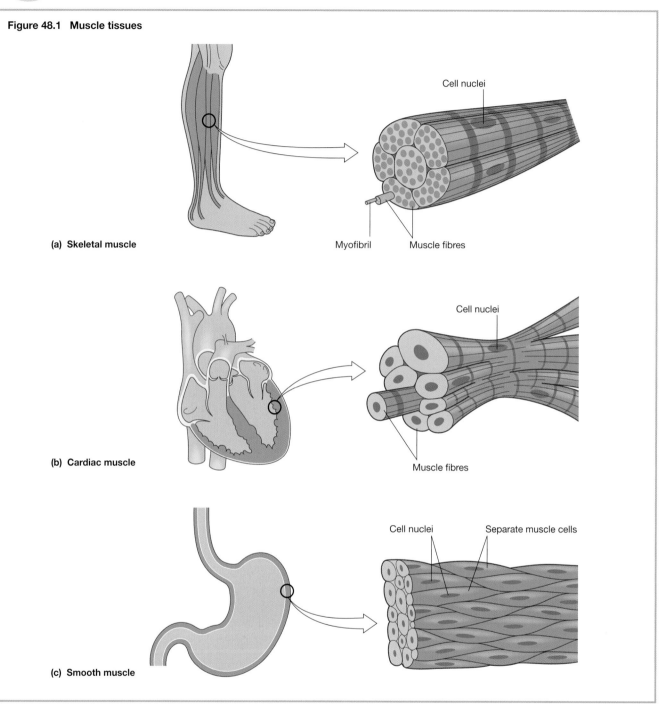

Figure 48.1   Muscle tissues

(a) **Skeletal muscle**

Cell nuclei

Myofibril   Muscle fibres

(b) **Cardiac muscle**

Cell nuclei

Muscle fibres

(c) **Smooth muscle**

Cell nuclei   Separate muscle cells

Muscles

The bones provide the framework for the body as well as providing leverage; however it is the muscles that pull the bones, muscles can only pull they cannot push, the bones cannot move body parts. Muscles contract and move the viscera and the blood vessels, cardiac muscle makes the heart beat. Energy is turned into locomotion by the muscles, helping to drive the body. Without muscles we would not be able to do anything, each time we move, we blink the eyelids, we swallow our food, we inhale and exhale, we smile or frown, muscle is involved. Muscle tissue generates heat as it contracts. Much of this chapter will concentrate on skeletal muscle.

Muscle tissue

There are three types of muscle tissue: skeletal, cardiac and smooth (see Figure 48.1).

Skeletal muscle tissue

This is made up of long single striated fibres. The fibres vary in length from a few centimetres to 40 cm. It has many nuclei at the margin of a cell.

This muscle is voluntary – it can be made to relax or contract as a result of conscious effort.

Skeletal muscle tissue is, as the name suggests, found in the skeletal muscles. The function of the majority of skeletal muscles is to move bones of the skeleton.

The function of skeletal muscle is to produce movement, maintain posture, produce heat and act in a protective manner.

Skeletal muscles are surrounded by connective tissue with a good nerve and blood supply. In the case of skeletal muscle, the individual cells (the fibres), are ordinarily long and thin, they become shorter and fatter under stimulus and have the ability to take a tremendous pulling power. When the stimulus has passed, the muscle relaxes, returning to its original shape.

The sarcolemma is the muscle cell, the cytoplasm is the sarcoplasm. The tubules begin at the sarcolemma extending into the sarcoplasm permitting the rapid distribution to contract throughout the muscle fibre. Muscle fibre contains myofibrils which shorten and are responsible for contraction, they consist of bundles of filaments made up of actin and myosin and organised into functional units called scarcomeres; actin filaments are thick and myosin are thin, thick filaments lie at the centre of the sarcomere and the thin filaments at either end. The Z line separates the sarcomere and the M line is in the middle. Actin and myosin filaments are jointed by cross bridges, during contraction the cross bridges engage and re-engage resulting in shortening. Calcium is released by a number of structures promoting muscle contraction. Each fibre is surrounded by a layer of endomysium joined in bundles forming fascicles, each of these are covered in perimysium.

The structure that permits the nerve impulse to initiate contraction is called the neuromuscular junction (NMJ). Each muscle fibre has one NMJ where the axon of the neuron joins the fibre. At the terminal end of the axon, closest to the motor endplate, the nerve and the motor endplate (not in direct contact) are separated by the synaptic cleft. The muscle is activated as a result of chemical transmission, the transmitter is acetyl choline contained in the axon; this then bonds to receptors that are located on the motor endplate.

Depolarisation of the sarcolemma occurs and the action potential spreads across the sarcolemma down the transverse tubules into the interior of the cells of the triads. Calcium is then released and muscle contracts.

Cardiac muscle tissue

These are branched striated fibres; usually this type of muscle has only one centrally located nucleus. Each end is attached by transverse thickenings of plasma membrane containing desmosomes and gap junctions. The desmosomes bolster tissue and hold fibres together as forceful contraction occurs. The gap junctions allow for rapid conduction of electrical signals in the heart. This type of muscle is involuntary; the contractions are not consciously controlled.

This muscle is found only in the walls of the heart.

Cardiac muscle functions in order to pump blood throughout the body.

Smooth muscle tissue

This is made of nonstriated involuntary fibres and contains a single, centrally based nucleus. Gap junctions are present connecting many individual fibres in some smooth muscle tissues; this permits powerful contractions of many muscle fibres in a unified manner, for example, in the iris of the eye, the walls of hollow organs, the blood vessels, stomach, intestines, urinary bladder and the uterus. Smooth muscle fibres contract separately as is the case with skeletal muscle.

Smooth muscle tissue provides movement, wave-like movement such as occurs with the propulsion of food as it travels through the gastrointestinal tract, contraction of the stomach and the urinary bladder.

Properties of muscle tissue

There are four properties of muscle tissue:

1 excitability (irritability) – the ability to receive and respond to stimuli via generation of an electrical pulse which results in contraction of the muscle cells;
2 contractility – ability to shorten;
3 extensibility – ability to be stretched or extended;
4 elasticity – ability of a muscle fibre to recoil and resume its resting length.

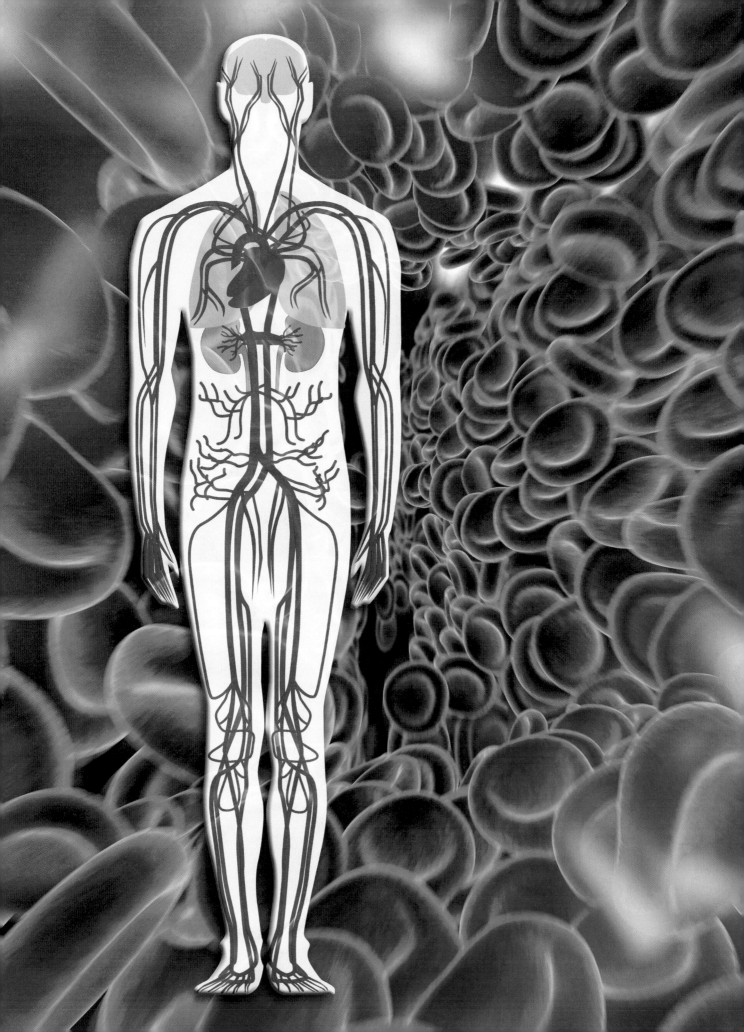

The skin

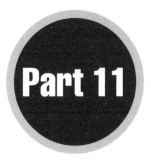
Part 11

49 The skin layers

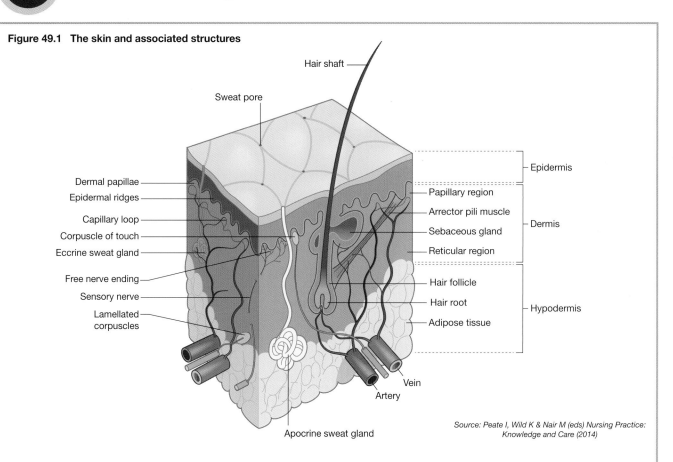

Figure 49.1 The skin and associated structures

Hair shaft

Sweat pore

Dermal papillae
Epidermal ridges
Capillary loop
Corpuscle of touch
Eccrine sweat gland
Free nerve ending
Sensory nerve
Lamellated corpuscles

Apocrine sweat gland

Epidermis

Papillary region
Arrector pili muscle
Sebaceous gland
Reticular region

Dermis

Hair follicle
Hair root
Adipose tissue

Hypodermis

Vein
Artery

Source: Peate I, Wild K & Nair M (eds) Nursing Practice: Knowledge and Care (2014)

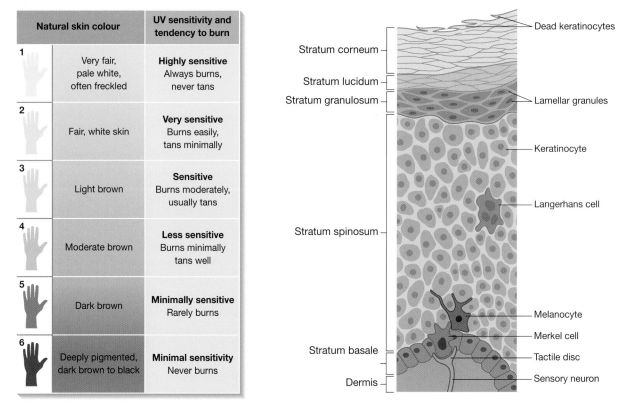

Figure 49.2 Skin types

Natural skin colour		UV sensitivity and tendency to burn
1	Very fair, pale white, often freckled	**Highly sensitive** Always burns, never tans
2	Fair, white skin	**Very sensitive** Burns easily, tans minimally
3	Light brown	**Sensitive** Burns moderately, usually tans
4	Moderate brown	**Less sensitive** Burns minimally tans well
5	Dark brown	**Minimally sensitive** Rarely burns
6	Deeply pigmented, dark brown to black	**Minimal sensitivity** Never burns

Figure 49.3 The layers of the epidermis

Stratum corneum
Stratum lucidum
Stratum granulosum

Stratum spinosum

Stratum basale

Dermis

Dead keratinocytes
Lamellar granules
Keratinocyte
Langerhans cell
Melanocyte
Merkel cell
Tactile disc
Sensory neuron

Anatomy and Physiology for Nurses at a Glance, First Edition. Ian Peate and Muralitharan Nair. © 2015 John Wiley & Sons, Ltd. Published 2015 by John Wiley & Sons, Ltd.
Companion website: www.ataglanceseries.com/nursing/anatomy

The skin

The skin (also called the integumentary system) is the largest organ of the body, it accounts for approximately 15% of the total adult body weight and it is composed of specialist cells and structures. The skin performs a number of essential functions; these include protecting the person against external physical, chemical and biological attack, it also prevents the loss of excess water loss from the body and plays a key a role in thermoregulation. The skin is continuous, with the mucous membranes that line the surface of the body.

The skin and its derivatives, for example, the hair, nails, sweat and oil glands make up the integumentary system (see Figure 49.1), it is composed of three layers:

- the epidermis
- the dermis
- subcutaneous tissue (hypodermis).

Throughout the body the skin's characteristics vary; for instance, the head contains more hair follicles than anywhere else, while the soles of the feet contain none. The thickness of the layers of the skin varies and this depends on where it is located on the body. The eyelids have the thinnest layer of the epidermis, this measures less than 0.1 mm, however the palms of the hands and soles of the feet have the thickest epidermal layer, this measures approximately 1.5 mm. On the back the dermis is at its thickest here, it is around 30–40 times as thick as the overlying epidermis. Skin type is another characteristic (see Figure 49.2).

The skin is constantly renewed. In relation to the other organs of the body, the skin can uncover various dysfunctions or pathologies.

There are four types of tissues in the skin: the epidermis that covers the surface of the body; connective tissue, this is made of protein fibres – it is tough and flexible; muscle in the skin interacts with hairs responding to various stimuli including heat and fright; and nervous tissue enables us to detect external stimuli such as pain and pressure.

The layers of the skin

The epidermis

The epidermis is the thinner and more superficial layer of the skin, made up of four types of cell. The keratinocytes are the most common type of skin cells; these cells produce keratin which is a fibrous protein that helps protect the epidermis. Keratin provides strength to skin, hair and nails. They are formed in the deep, basal cell layer of the skin gradually migrating upwards, where they become squamous cells prior to reaching the surface of the skin over the course of about four weeks. Melanocytes are responsible for synthesising the brown pigment, melanin. Pigmentation is extremely heritable, regulated by genetic, environmental and endocrine factors that regulate the amount, type and the distribution of melanin in the skin, hair and eyes. Melanocytes are cells located in the lower part of the epidermis, just above the dermis. It is melanin that gives colour to the skin, hair and parts of the eye. Melanin also plays an important role in protecting the skin from the harmful radiation produced by ultraviolet (UV) radiation; it is an important defence system of the skin against harmful factors. The Langerhan cells are

associated with immune response; they regulate immune reactions in the skin. These cells work by ingesting antigens that get into the skin, presenting them to cells of the immune system. The dendritic Langerhans cells originate in the bone marrow. They then migrate to the epidermis where they form a regularly arranged network that can reach a density of approximately 700 to 800 cells per square millimetre. The touch receptor cells – the Merkel cells – participate in the sense of touch and are located primarily in the basal layer of the epidermis. There is much variation in the density of the Merkel cells; the fingertips and the plantar aspects of the toes have a far greater density than any other part of the body.

There are five separate sub-layers of the epidermis:

1 Stratum corneum: the outermost layer has 25–30 layers of dead flat keratinocytes. Lamellar granules provide water repellent action and are continuously shed and replaced.

2 Stratum lucidum: this is only found in the fingertips, palms of hands and soles of feet. This layer is made up of 3–5 layers of flat dead keratinocytes.

3 Stratum granulosum: is made up of 3–5 layers of keratinocytes and is the site of keratin formation, keratohyalin gives it its granular appearance.

4 Stratum spinosum: appears as if covered in thornlike spikes, providing the skin with strength and flexibility.

5 Stratum basale: this is the deepest layer, made up of a single layer of cuboidal or columnar cells. Cells produced in this layer are constantly dividing and move up to the surface (See Figure 49.3).

The dermis

This layer is composed of connective tissue; blood vessels, nerves, glands and hair follicles, collagen and elastic fibres help with strength and elasticity. The cell types in the epidermis include the kerinocytes, melanocytes, Langerhans cells and Merkel cells. The functions of the adipocytes include sensitivity to insulin and the ability to produce and secrete adipocyte-specific endocrine hormones regulating energy homeostasis in other tissues; they are critical regulators of whole-body metabolism. Macrophages with fibroblasts play a central role in wound healing.

The two main divisions of the dermal layer are the papillary region in the superficial layer of the dermis, made up of loose areolar connective tissue with elastic fibres, and the dermal papillae – these are fingerlike structures invading the epidermis containing capillaries or Meissner corpuscles which respond to touch.

The subcutaneous tissues

Sometimes called the subcutis or the hypodermis, this is the deepest layer of the skin.

Subcutaneous tissue is an important line of defence, composed of an insulating layer of fat and blood vessels. The size of this layer varies throughout the body and from person to person. The fat in the subcutaneous layer offers protection to the organs and bones helping maintain body temperature, working with the blood vessels to keep temperature normal and consistent. The sweat glands in this layer are also important in thermoregulation. As the body ages, subcutaneous tissue begins to thin out.

50 The skin appendages

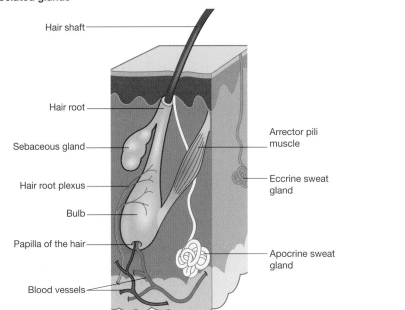

Hair shaft

Hair root

Sebaceous gland

Hair root plexus

Bulb

Papilla of the hair

Blood vessels

Arrector pili muscle

Eccrine sweat gland

Apocrine sweat gland

Source: Peate I, Wild K & Nair M (eds) Nursing Practice: Knowledge and Care (2014)

Figure 50.2 The nails

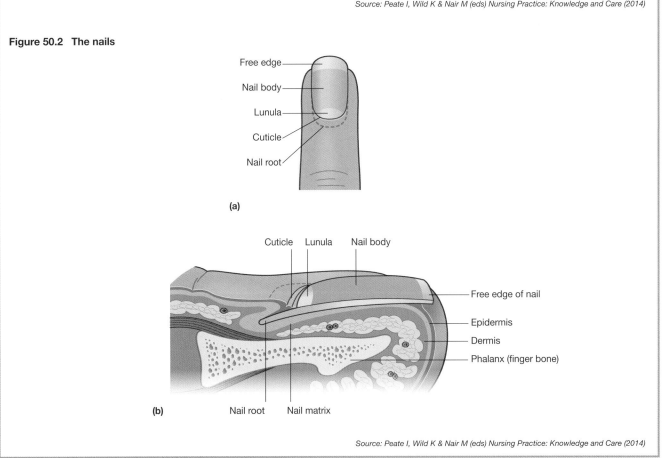

Free edge

Nail body

Lunula

Cuticle

Nail root

(a)

Cuticle   Lunula   Nail body

Free edge of nail

Epidermis

Dermis

Phalanx (finger bone)

(b)   Nail root   Nail matrix

Source: Peate I, Wild K & Nair M (eds) Nursing Practice: Knowledge and Care (2014)

The appendages of the skin are sometimes also referred to as the derivatives of the integument. The appendages include the hair, the nails and the glands.

The dermal appendages

The hair

The hair provides a variety of functions and these include protection, thermoregulation and sensing light touch. Hair is composed of a variety of columns of dead, elongated keratinised cells that are bound together by extracellular proteins. There are two main sections associated with the hair:
- The shaft: this is the superficial portion that extends out of the skin.
- The root: this portion penetrates into the dermis.

The hair follicle is a small blind-ended tubular structure consisting of five concentric layers of epithelial cells extending from the dermis through to the epidermis containing the hair root. At the base of the hair follicle is a bulbous expansion, an onion-shaped structure (a bulb) that is called the papilla of the hair and the matrix contained within the bulb produces new hair. The sebaceous and the apocrine skin glands have ducts that lead into the hair follicle.

During hair formation the inner three layers undergo keratinisation and the outer two layers form an epithelial sheath. At age three months hairs begin to appear over the eyebrow and the upper lip. There are three stages of hair growth: the anagen phase, this is the fast growing phase; the involution phase is called the catangen phase; and the third phase is the telogen phase, this is the rest phase.

There are three specific types of hair: lanugo hairs – these are foetal hairs, vellus hairs – infant hairs and fine body hair. The final type – the coarse hair type – is called terminal hair. The distribution of the hair differs between the sexes after puberty has occurred.

The arrector pili muscles are small muscles that are attached to hair follicles (see Figure 50.1). This muscle extends from the dermal coat of the hair follicle to the papillary layer of the dermis. It is this muscle that causes goose bumps (the cholinergic sympathetic supply). The portion where the arrector pili muscle inserts is called the bulge area and it is thought that at this location the stem cells that are responsible for the regeneration of the hair follicle are located.

The nail

The nails participate in grasping and handling of small things. Nails are highly versatile tools that protect the fingertip, contribute to tactile sensation by acting as a counterforce to the fingertip pad and aid in peripheral thermoregulation via glomus bodies located in the nail bed and matrix (see Figure 50.2).

Nails are plates of very tightly packed, hard, keratinised epidermal cells; they develop from the thickened areas of epidermis located at the tips of fingers, thumbs and toes known as nail fields. The nail fields travel on to the dorsal surface surrounded on both sides by folds of epidermis known as nail folds. They are usually located on the dorsal aspect of each distal phalanx. The nail consists of a nail root, this is the portion of the nail under the skin, a nail body, the visible pink aspect of the nail, the white crescent located at the base of the nail is called the lunula, the hyponychium secures the nail to the finger, the cuticle or eponychium is a narrow band around the proximal edge of the nail, and a free edge – this is the white end that can extend past the finger.

The almost transparent nail plate combined with the thin epithelium of the nail bed provide a useful way of observing the amount of oxygen present in the blood by revealing the colour of blood in the dermal vessels.

Nails are growing continuously; however, the rate at which they grow slows down as a person ages and if there is evidence of poor circulation. Fingernails grow faster than toenails, the growth rate of a fingernail is said to be in the region of 1–3 mm every four weeks, toenails grow about 1 mm per month and take 12–18 months to be completely replaced. Complete nail plate growth may take approximately six months. There are some factors that will increase the rate of the growth; these will include longer digits, summer months, young persons (those less than 30 years) and if the person bites their nails.

The glands

The glands play a key role in the regulation of body temperature. There are three main types of glands associated with the skin:
1 the sebaceous gland,
2 the sudoriferous glands,
3 the ceruminous glands.

The sebaceous glands

These are oil-secreting glands located in the dermis which secrete sebum. Sebaceous glands are found over most of the surface of the body but are not present on the palms of the hands or the soles of the feet. Sebum helps to prevent hairs from becoming too dry and brittle, preventing the skin from becoming too dry (by preventing excessive evaporation of water from the skin's surface) it also restricts the growth and development of certain bacteria.

The sudoriferous glands

The sudoriferous glands (these are also known as sweat glands) are divided into two main types. Eccrine glands' ducts terminate at a sweat pore at the outer surface of the epidermis; these are the most common type and their key function is to regulate body temperature by evaporation. Eccrine glands are located throughout the skin except for the margins of the lips, the tympanic membrane and the nail beds of the finger and toenails. Apocrine glands are responsible for 'cold sweats' that are associated with stressful experiences, their ducts open in hair follicles, they are found in the axillae, the pubic regions and the areola of the breasts.

The ceruminous glands

These glands are located in subcutaneous tissue below the dermis; they secrete cerumen (ear wax) into the ear canal or sebaceous glands. Cerumen, along with the hairs in the outer ear, protects the ear from particles originating outside of the body – for example, dust, fine sand, or similar – getting into the ear itself. Cerumen provides a sticky barrier preventing many such particles from going further into the ear.

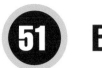

51 Epithelialisation

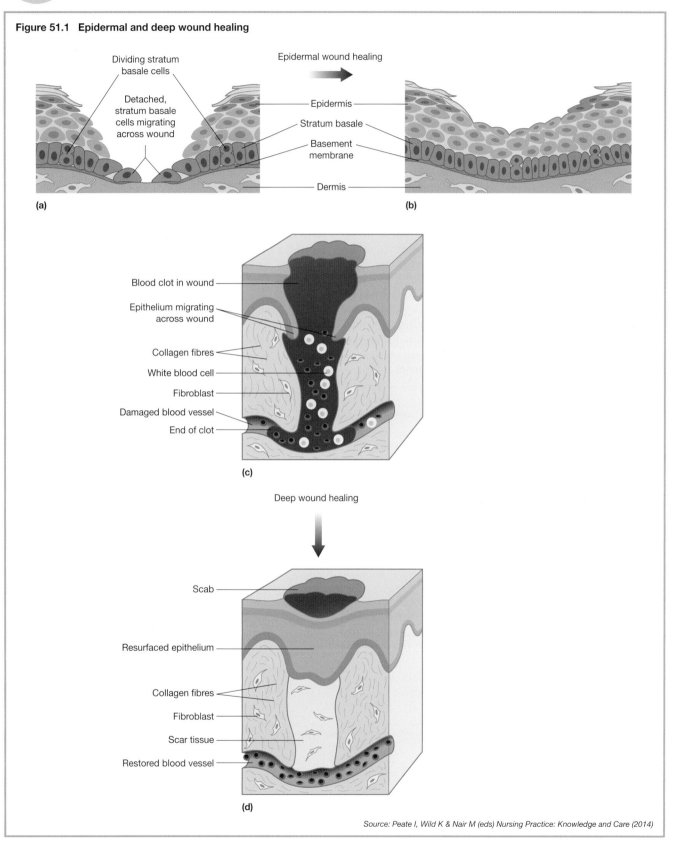

Figure 51.1 Epidermal and deep wound healing

Dividing stratum basale cells

Detached, stratum basale cells migrating across wound

Epidermal wound healing

Epidermis

Stratum basale

Basement membrane

Dermis

(a)

(b)

Blood clot in wound

Epithelium migrating across wound

Collagen fibres

White blood cell

Fibroblast

Damaged blood vessel

End of clot

(c)

Deep wound healing

Scab

Resurfaced epithelium

Collagen fibres

Fibroblast

Scar tissue

Restored blood vessel

(d)

Source: Peate I, Wild K & Nair M (eds) Nursing Practice: Knowledge and Care (2014)

Epithelialisation

This is the body's physiological response to healing in its attempt to restore and maintain homeostasis. Epithelialisation usually occurs in response to tissue damage; for example, after a wound has occurred.

Wounds

A wound is a breakdown in the protective functions provided by the skin where there is loss of continuity of the epithelium; this may or may not include the underlying connective tissue – for example, the muscle, bone or nerve – after an injury to the skin has occurred that may be caused by surgery, direct trauma, a cut, chemicals, heat/cold, friction/shear force, pressure or as a result of pathology (for example, cancer). Wounds can be described in a number of ways; by the cause (aetiology), anatomical location, whether the wound is acute or chronic, by the method of closure (primary, secondary or delayed closure), by presenting symptoms or by the appearance of the predominant tissue types in the wound bed. The goal in wound management is to restore structure and function and to enhance the cosmetic appearance as quickly as possible. Injuries that occur to the epidermis are epidermal wounds; deeper wounds penetrate and enter the dermis.

How wounds heal

When a wound has occurred (damage to the skin) this then sets in action a range of activities that set out to achieve the goals associated with wound management and to re-establish skin integrity. There are a number of ways in which wounds can heal and they follow a predictable order of events. The wound has only two mechanisms by which it can heal: tissue regeneration or tissue repair.

All wounds, cutaneous or skin, heal by two independent methods, contraction and epithelialisation.

Contraction occurs as a wound heals, producing a bed of granulation tissues causing the edges of the wound to contract. This eventually covers the surface of the wound.

Epithelialisation is a complex process that is associated with cell proliferation. As cells proliferate they migrate covering the surface of the cutaneous defect.

The epidermis has the capacity to regenerate identical cells; in superficial damage when the basal layer of the dermis is still intact, normal anatomical structure and function is restored quickly.

When the injury extends deeper, penetrating the dermis and causing damage to some of the intricate structures such as the hair follicles, sweat glands, nerve and blood vessels, then there are more complex biological processes required to carry out tissue repair. The anatomical structure and function (depending on the extent of damage) may not be restored. Figure 51.1 shows epidermal and deep wound healing.

Types of wound healing
Primary closure

Sometimes called healing by primary intention, healing follows minimal damage to tissues where the borders of the wound are in close opposition. This involves re-epithelialisation, the outer layer closes over the wound. Cells grow in from the margins of the wound and out from epithelial cells, lining the hair follicles and sweat glands.

Inflammation occurs where the surfaces have been cut, blood clot formation and cell debris fill the breach between the edges. Phagocytes begin to remove the clots and cell debris, encouraging fibroblast activity. Collagen fibres are secreted by the fibroblasts, beginning to bring the surfaces together.

Epithelial cells proliferate across the wound; the epidermis meets and grows upwards, ceasing when full thickness has occurred. The clot formed becomes a scab.

Wounds where the boarders are in close opposition (well-approximated) are those that can be closely aligned, for example, a surgical incision. In the case of a surgical incision the edges of the wound are mechanically brought together without tension. Closure can occur using butterfly sutures (adhesive strips), sutures, glue (skin adhesives), clips or staples. As there is no loss of tissue, and if there is no risk of infection, the healing process in this case is quick. Often these types of wound heal in 4 to 21 days and result in minimal scarring and best aesthetic appearance.

Secondary closure

Wounds that heal by secondary closure, where primary closure is not possible, may involve some degree of tissue loss and the margins of the wound cannot be approximated. A wound's depth can be described as partial thickness or full thickness. As wounds heal by secondary intention, the wound fills with granulation tissue and re-epithelialisation occurs, principally from the wound edges, and eventually a scar forms. These wounds take longer to heal with scarring.

Delayed primary closure

Sometimes this is known as tertiary wound closure. Wounds in this category are intentionally kept open allowing local conditions such as oedema or infection to abate or to allow the elimination of exudate. As conditions improve these wounds are later closed using sutures or other procedures.

Wound closure

This occurs when a number of processes combine. These include granulation, contraction and epithelisation.

The final stage of wound healing is epithelialisation. Epithelialisation occurs when the germinal layer of the epidermis (stratum basale) responds to chemical signals to proliferate and migrate across the granulation tissue with the intention of forming a new layer of epidermal cells. When this occurs a new basement membrane and dermo-epidermal junction is created and the neoepidermis maintains proliferation and differentiates into the stratified, cornified epithelium (stratum corneum) of normal skin. There is active division, migration and maturation of epidermal cells from the wound edges across the open wound. Speedy epithelialisation is dependent upon a source of epidermal cells, a wound bed that is composed of healthy granulation tissue and a favourable wound microenvironment. Epithelialisation progresses depending upon the size of the wound and how it changes over time.

52 Granulation

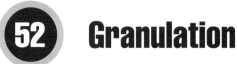

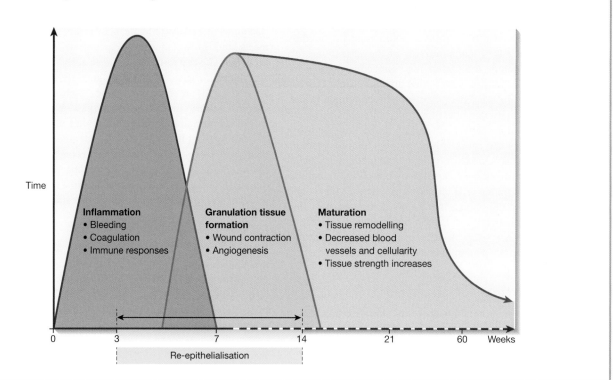

Figure 52.1 Summary of wound healing events

Time

Inflammation
• Bleeding
• Coagulation
• Immune responses

Granulation tissue formation
• Wound contraction
• Angiogenesis

Maturation
• Tissue remodelling
• Decreased blood vessels and cellularity
• Tissue strength increases

0   3   7   14   21   60   Weeks

Re-epithelialisation

Granulation is an essential physiological requirement needed for wound healing, others include epithelisation (see Chapter 51) and contraction. Figure 52.1 provides a summary of wound healing events.

Granulation tissue

Tissue granulation occurs in the proliferative phase of the process of wound healing, during which new, healthy tissue reforms and rebuilds the area of the wound. Granulation tissue is tissue that is composed of a newly formed wound matrix – containing collagen, matrix proteins and proteoglycans – that forms at the site of an injury. This collagen matrix offers the scaffolding (structural strength) into which new capillaries grow. During granulation the skin cells are most active, granulation tissue is actively growing connective tissue.

Angiogenesis (the creation of new blood vessels and in this instance capillary formation) supports the growth of new connective tissue along with the nourishment of macrophages and the collagen-secreting fibroblasts. The presence of hyaluronic acid within the extracellular matrix stimulates the production of cytokines, such as transforming growth factor (TGF), that act on the macrophages to encourage angiogenesis. Macrophages that migrate to the wound are further stimulated into angiogenesis as they come into contact with the hypoxic wound environment that has been caused by damage to the blood supply when injury occurred.

When a wound begins the granulation process, this indicates that the body is commencing to rebuild after the injury. Granulation tissue is a highly fibrous tissue that is typically pink as the body produces numerous small capillaries to provide a rich supply of oxygen and nutrients as well as assisting in the removal of waste. Granulation tissue appears bumpy and uneven. As the process begins granulation tissue may appear reddened and irritated, as a result of the numerous blood vessels it contains.

The subsequent granulation tissue present in the wound is red in colour and this is often described as granular or grainy in its appearance. The tissue eventually fills up the injury site and a scar may appear; this fades over time.

The ability of injured tissue to restore itself is contingent on the amount of damage as well as the regenerative capability of the injured tissue. In large open wounds, for example, the parenchyma (these are the cells that make up the functioning part of the skin) and the stroma (the supporting connective tissue) become active in tissue repair.

Tissue repair

The success of tissue repair is based on a number of factors and these include nutrition and blood supply. The process of healing demands much nutritional support and draws on the body's nutritional stores. As the majority of structural components of tissue are protein it is essential therefore that the diet contains a sufficient amount of protein. There are also a number of vitamins that play a central role in the healing of wounds and the repair of tissue. When there are deficiencies in vitamins, minerals and trace elements wound healing will be negatively influenced. Under the direct influence of vitamin C are collagen synthesis, the development of the delicate fibrils usually present in collagen fibres of connective tissues (this is called fibrillogenesis) and angiogenesis. Vitamin B is directly responsible for the production of protein, formation of antibodies, development of granulation tissue and epithelialisation. Vitamin A has a central role to play in angiogenesis, macrophage mobility and chemotaxis, this vitamin also manages some of the negative effects radiation has on wound healing.

Haemoglobin synthesis involves iron and as such oxygenation trace elements such as copper and zinc are required for encouraging collagen formation and epithelisation.

Blood circulation is essential for the transportation of oxygen, nutrients, antibodies and other cells involved in defending the body to the site of injury where granulation and tissue repair is to take place.

Blood removes bacteria, foreign bodies and debris that would otherwise impact on the healing process.

When a significant amount of granulation does occur, it usually leaves a visible and wide scar as a result of the difference between the new and the old tissue.

The final phase of wound healing is the remodelling phase, when the new tissue fully integrates with the old tissue. This phase may take weeks, months, or years depending on the severity of the wound; in many cases, complete remodelling does not occur and scars remain behind.

Over-granulation

In some instances an excess of granulation tissue (also called hypergranulation) may be produced which impacts on migrating keratinocytes. The presence of such tissue prevents epithelial migration across the wound, which delays wound healing. Granulation continues even when granulation tissue is level with the surrounding skin.

Hypergranulation tissue is usually seen as a pale or light purple uneven mass that rises above the level of the skin. Excessive and extended stimulation of fibroblasts and angiogenesis appear as mounds of granulation tissue that bleed easily and ooze haemoserous exudate. Over-granulation can interfere with the rate of wound healing.

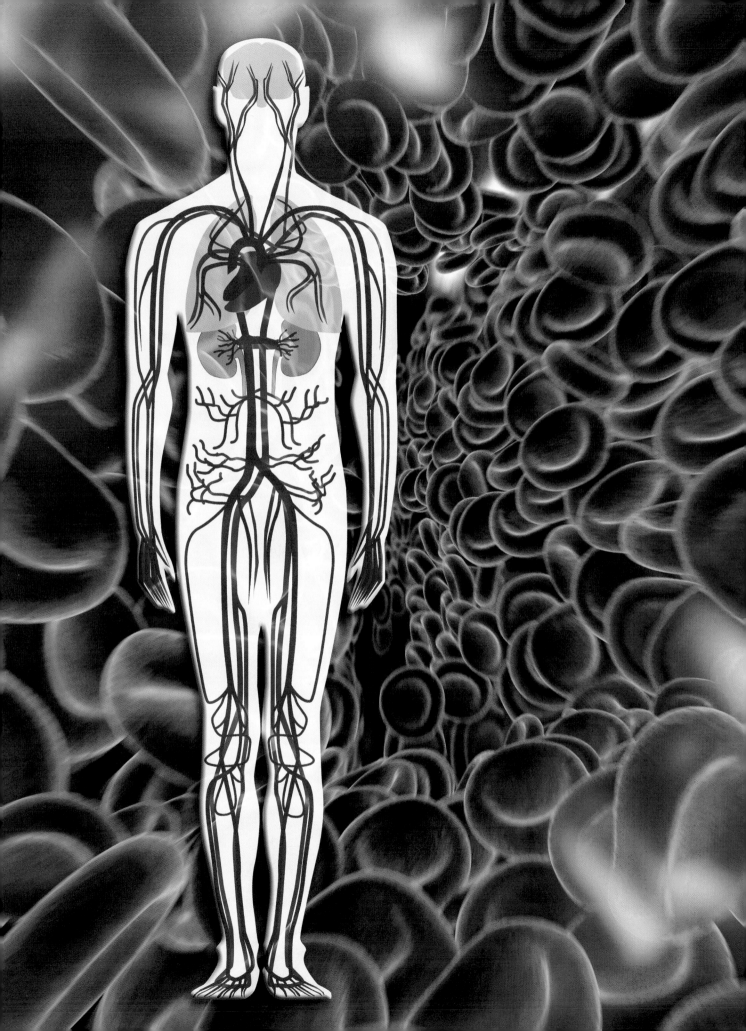

The senses

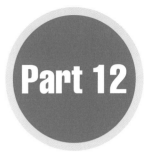

Part 12

Chapters

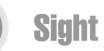

53 Sight

Figure 53.1   The eye

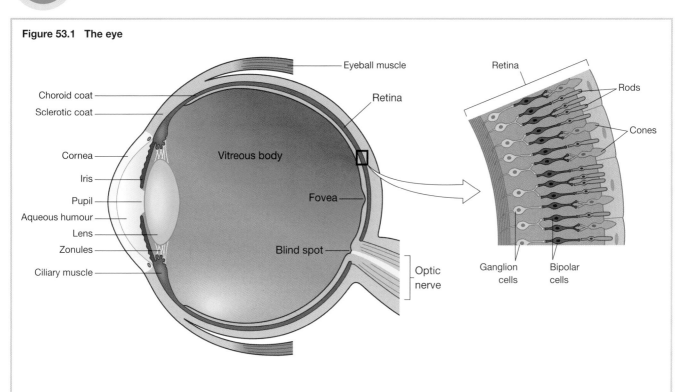

Table 53.1   The eye

Structures that protect the eye	Anterior aspect of the eye	Posterior aspect of the eye	The visual system pathways to the brain
• Orbit • Eye lids • Eye lashes and eyebrows • Lacrimal apparatus • Sclera	• Cornea • Aqueous humour • Iris • Lens and ciliary muscle	• Retina • Vitreous humour	• Optic nerves and optic tracts • Visual cortex

Figure 53.2   The lacrimal apparatus

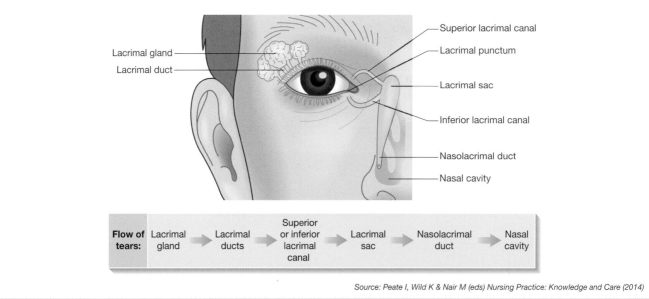

Source: Peate I, Wild K & Nair M (eds) Nursing Practice: Knowledge and Care (2014)

Anatomy and Physiology for Nurses at a Glance, First Edition. Ian Peate and Muralitharan Nair. © 2015 John Wiley & Sons, Ltd. Published 2015 by John Wiley & Sons, Ltd.
Companion website: www.ataglanceseries.com/nursing/anatomy

There is no agreement as to how many special senses there are. In this part of the text there will be reference to four senses. The special senses are smell, taste, vision and hearing (including equilibrium). They are known as the special senses because their sensory receptors are located within relatively large sensory organs located in the head, the nose, tongue, eyes and ears. The skin is sometimes considered a sense organ, touch is not considered a special sense but a generalised one (see Part 11: The skin).

Sight

The eye permits us to see and understand shapes, colours and dimensions of objects by processing the light they reflect or emit. The eye is capable of detecting bright light or dim light, it is a complex structure designed to gather a significant amount of information concerning the environment. See Table 53.1 for the areas related to the eye.

The eye consists of the cornea, iris, pupil, lens and retina (this houses the light-sensitive photoreceptors) (Figure 53.1).

The orbit

Two orbits protect the eyes located at the front of the skull, with a wider opening anteriorly narrowing to a small opening posteriorly where the optic nerve exits connecting to the visual pathways and brain.

The eye lids, eye lashes and eye brows

External to the eyeball these structures provide protection. Other protective structures include the conjunctiva, lacrimal apparatus and extrinsic eye muscles.

Eyelids are thin, loose folds of skin covering the anterior eye, protecting the eye from foreign bodies and excessive light, they also spread tears by blinking. They contain the puncta through which tears flow. Eyebrows provide shade, keeping perspiration and other debris away from the eyes. Eyelashes protect from foreign particles acting as sensors, they are short hairs projecting from the top and bottom borders of the eyelids. An unexpected touch initiates the blinking reflex.

The lacrimal apparatus

The lacrimal apparatus (see Figure 53.2) produces and drains lacrimal fluid. The surface of the eye is continuously bathed in tears predominantly secreted by the lacrimal gland, conjunctival secretions are also added. These structures secrete, distribute and drain, cleaning and moistening the eye's surface.

Fluid is pumped throughout the system each time blinking occurs. Tears are drained away via the nasolacrimal system they have antimicrobial properties.

The sclera

This is derived from interwoven collagen fibrils of varying widths within ground substance maintained by fibroblasts. Made up from three layers of varying thickness.

The cornea

Transparent to light, it does not contain blood vessels and is approximately 11 mm in diameter and 500 μm thick in the centre. The cornea is more curved than the rest of the globe. With the lens it transmits and focuses light into the eye, and protects the inner ocular structures.

The aqueous humour

This is a transparent fluid filling the anterior chamber of the eye, providing oxygen and nutrients to the lens and cornea. Between the cornea and the front surface of the crystalline lens is the aqueous humour; continuously filtering out of blood vessels in the ciliary processes of the ciliary body. The aqueous is a part of the optical pathway of the eye.

The iris

The coloured aspect of the eyeball, shaped like a flattened doughnut, controls light levels inside the eye similar to the aperture on a camera. The round opening in the centre is the pupil. A number of tiny muscles embedded in the iris dilate and constrict pupil size.

The circular sphincter muscle (innervated by the parasympathetic system) lies around the very edge of the pupil, causing the pupil to constrict in bright light. The radial dilator muscle (innervated by the parasympathetic system) runs radially through the iris, dilating the eye in dim lighting.

The lens and ciliary muscle

The lens is posterior to the pupil and the iris, it is a transparent structure, changing its shape in order to increase or decrease the amount of refracting power applied to light coming into the eye. The lens provides the remaining variable focusing power and serves to further refine the focus, permitting the eye to focus on objects at different distances.

An elastic extracellular matrix, the capsule surrounds the lens providing a smooth optical surface, it is an anchor for the suspension of the lens within the eye. A meshwork of nonelastic microfibrils, or 'zonules', anchor into the capsule close to the equator of the lens connecting into ciliary muscle. Ciliary muscle is part of the ciliary body, divided into ciliary muscle, ciliary processes and pars plana.

The retina

Mostly this is a transparent thin tissue designed to capture photons of light and initiate processing of the image by the brain. Average thickness of the retina is 250 μm and it consists of 10 layers.

There are two types of receptors: rods and cones: The outer segment contains light sensitive visual pigment molecules – opsins – in stacked disks (rods) or invaginations (cones). Cones provide the ability to discern colour and the ability to see fine detail, they are more concentrated in the central retina. Rods are mainly responsible for peripheral vision; vision under low light conditions, and are more prevalent in the mid-peripheral and peripheral retina.

The visual system pathways to the brain

The optic nerves meet at the optic chiasma. At the optic chiasma, axons from the medial half of each retina cross to the opposite side, forming pairs of axons from each eye – the left and right optic tracts. The crossing of the axons results in each optic tract carrying information from both eyes, the left carries visual information from the lateral half of the retina of the left eye and the medial half of the retina of the right eye, whereas the right one carries visual information from the lateral half of the retina of the right eye and the medial half of the retina of the left eye.

The visual cortex

Located in the occipital lobe of the brain, where the final processing of the neural signals from the retina takes place and vision occurs. The occipital lobe is at the most posterior portion of the brain, with six separate areas in the visual cortex.

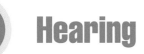

Hearing

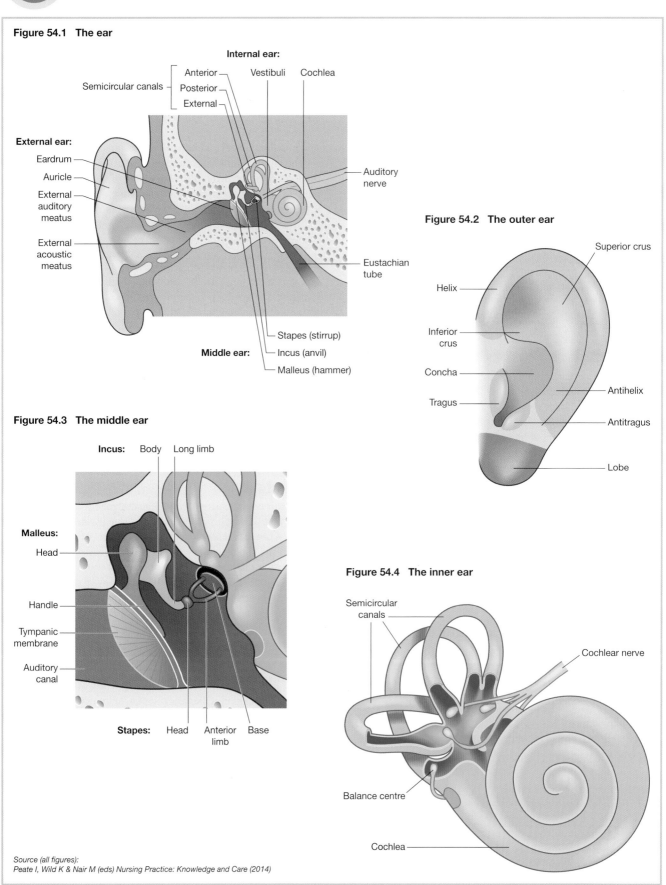

Figure 54.1   The ear

Internal ear:
Semicircular canals
Anterior
Posterior
External
Vestibuli
Cochlea

External ear:
Eardrum
Auricle
External auditory meatus
External acoustic meatus

Auditory nerve

Eustachian tube

Stapes (stirrup)
Incus (anvil)
Malleus (hammer)
Middle ear:

Figure 54.2   The outer ear

Helix
Inferior crus
Concha
Tragus
Superior crus
Antihelix
Antitragus
Lobe

Figure 54.3   The middle ear

Incus: Body   Long limb

Malleus:
Head
Handle
Tympanic membrane
Auditory canal

Stapes: Head   Anterior limb   Base

Figure 54.4   The inner ear

Semicircular canals
Cochlear nerve
Balance centre
Cochlea

Source (all figures):
Peate I, Wild K & Nair M (eds) Nursing Practice: Knowledge and Care (2014)

Anatomy and Physiology for Nurses at a Glance, First Edition. Ian Peate and Muralitharan Nair. © 2015 John Wiley & Sons, Ltd. Published 2015 by John Wiley & Sons, Ltd.
Companion website: www.ataglanceseries.com/nursing/anatomy

Hearing

Sound represents a combination of waves generated by a vibrating sound source(s) propagated through the air until they reach the ear. Wave frequency corresponds to what is perceived as pitch, amplitude corresponds to the loudness or intensity of sound.

The ear

The ear has two key functions: to assist with balance (equilibrium) and to allow us to hear the sounds around us. The ear is composed of three sections (see Figure 54.1):

- outer (external)
- middle
- inner.

The outer (external ear)

This aspect of the ear assists with functions of the middle ear although it is not an anatomical part of it. The auricle and external acoustic meatus (external auditory canal) compose the external ear. The external ear functions to collect and amplify sound, which is transmitted to the middle ear. The asymmetric shape introduces delays in the path of sound assisting in sound localisation. See Figure 54.2.

The arterial supply is composed of the posterior auricular artery, the anterior auricular branch of the superficial temporal artery, and the occipital artery, which also contributes. Veins accompany corresponding named arteries.

The external ear is supplied by the auriculotemporal (fifth cranial) nerve and contributions from cranial nerves VII, IX and X and the great auricular nerve.

The middle ear

The key function of the middle ear (tympanic cavity) is that of bony conduction of sound via transference of sound waves in the air collected by the auricle to the fluid of the inner ear. The middle ear sits in the petrous portion of the temporal bone and is filled with air secondary to communication with the nasopharynx via the auditory (eustachian) tube (see Figure 54.3).

The middle ear extends from the tympanic membrane to the oval window containing the bony conduction elements of the ossicles. The walls of the tympanic cavity are complex with important associations.

Tympanic membrane

The tympanic membrane is an oval, thin, semi-transparent membrane separating the external and middle ear. Air vibrations collected by the auricle are transferred to the mobile tympanic membrane, which then transmits the sound to the ossicles. Multiple structures are contained within the tympanic cavity. Muscles, nerves, and the auditory tube occupy space within the tympanic cavity.

Ossicles

From the deep surface of the tympanic membrane to the oval window is a chain of movable bones, the ossicles, malleus (hammer), incus (anvil) and stapes (stirrup). These serve to transmit and amplify sound waves from the air to the perilymph of the internal ear.

Auditory tube

The auditory tube (eustachian tube) is the communication between the middle ear and the nasopharynx. It equalises pressure across the tympanic membrane.

The blood supply is derived from a number of arteries, primarily from the external and internal carotid. The middle ear is supplied by the auriculotemporal (Vth cranial) and tympanic (IXth cranial) nerves and by the auricular branch of the vagus.

The inner ear

The inner ear consists of a membranous 'labyrinth' encased in an osseous labyrinth. The vestibule and semicircular canals are associated with vestibular function (balance). The cochlea is concerned with hearing, this is a coiled tube (see Figure 54.4).

A layer of dense bone creates the surface outline of the inner ear. The walls of the bony labyrinth are continuous with the surrounding temporal bone. The inner aspects of the bony labyrinth closely follow the contours of the membranous labyrinth; a delicate, interconnected network of fluid-filled tubes where the receptors are found.

The walls of the bony labyrinth are made up of dense bone, apart from two small areas located close to the cochlear spiral. The round window consists of a thin, membranous partition separating the perilymph of the cochlear chambers from the air-filled middle ear. Collagen fibres connect the bony margins of the oval window at the base of the stapes.

Perilymph, which closely resembles cerebrospinal fluid, flows between the bony and membranous labyrinths. Endolymph is contained in the membranous labyrinth. These fluids are in separate compartments. The bony labyrinth can be subdivided into the vestibule, three semicircular canals and the cochlea.

The vestibule

This contains a pair of membranous sacs: the saccule and the utricle. Receptors here provide for sensations of gravity and linear acceleration.

The semicircular canals

These enclose the slender semicircular ducts. Receptors are stimulated when the head moves. The fluid-filled chambers within the vestibule are usually continuous with the semicircular canals.

The cochlea

A bony, spiral-shaped chamber, it contains the cochlear duct of the membranous labyrinth. The sense of hearing is provided by receptors within the cochlear duct. Two perilymph-filled chambers are on either side of the duct.

Blood supply to the inner ear

The internal auditory artery supplies the entire membranous labyrinth passing through the internal auditory meatus, dividing into three branches. The cochlear artery supplies the entire cochlea via the spiral arteries.

The organ of Corti

This is located in the cochlea and is referred to as the receptor organ of hearing. Hair cells within the organ of Corti sense mechanical forces (inner and the outer hair cells); 95% of the afferent fibres are from the inner hair cells, these are the sensory receptors communicating with neurons for the VIIIth cranial nerve, outer hair cells receive efferent input.

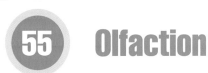

Olfaction

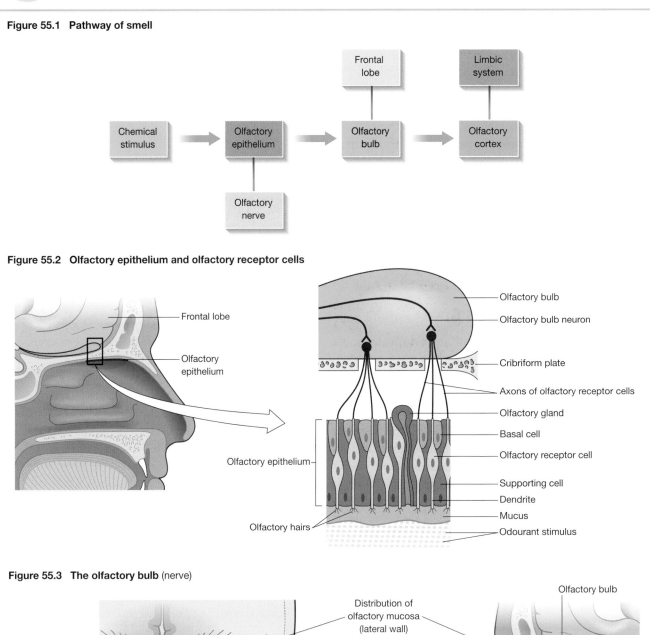

Figure 55.1 Pathway of smell

```
                                    Frontal              Limbic
                                     lobe                system

Chemical        Olfactory        Olfactory           Olfactory
stimulus   →    epithelium   →      bulb         →      cortex

                Olfactory
                  nerve
```

Figure 55.2 Olfactory epithelium and olfactory receptor cells

Frontal lobe

Olfactory epithelium

Olfactory bulb

Olfactory bulb neuron

Cribriform plate

Axons of olfactory receptor cells

Olfactory gland

Basal cell

Olfactory receptor cell

Supporting cell

Dendrite

Mucus

Odourant stimulus

Olfactory epithelium

Olfactory hairs

Figure 55.3 The olfactory bulb (nerve)

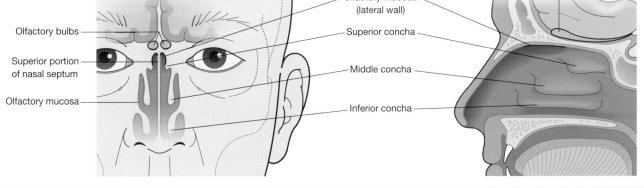

Distribution of
olfactory mucosa
(lateral wall)

Olfactory bulb

Olfactory bulbs

Superior concha

Superior portion
of nasal septum

Middle concha

Olfactory mucosa

Inferior concha

Anatomy and Physiology for Nurses at a Glance, First Edition. Ian Peate and Muralitharan Nair. © 2015 John Wiley & Sons, Ltd. Published 2015 by John Wiley & Sons, Ltd.
Companion website: www.ataglanceseries.com/nursing/anatomy

Olfaction, the sense of smell is (along with taste) a chemical sense. The sensations come from the interaction of molecules with smell receptors. Some smells can evoke strong emotional responses as the impulse for smell spreads to the limbic system (see Figure 55.1). When a person is constantly exposed to an odour, the perception of the odour will diminish and cease within minutes, the loss of perception only involves that specific odour.

With the sense of smell we are able to evaluate our environment taking in a large amount of information. We are always assessing the air that we inhale, this can alert us to possible dangers, for example, the presence of smoke. Smell also enables us to decipher other important information, such as the quality of food – if it's edible or potentially poisonous (rotten or gone off) as well as being able to identify the presence of another being it also influences social and sexual behaviour. Humans have an innate ability to detect bad, unpleasant, dangerous smells. The sense of smell is important for survival and the quality of life.

Physiology of olfaction

The nose contains between 10 and 100 million olfactory receptor neurons – which line the olfactory epithelium that lines the nasal mucosa in the nasal cavity – that are able to detect odours.

The olfactory system starts with olfactory receptor cells that are situated in the nasal epithelium of the nasal cavity (see Figure 55.2). Above this is a layer of protective bone. Axons of the olfactory receptor cells merge forming the olfactory nerves. The ends of the axons form spherical glomeruli, each of them receives input from the same olfactory receptor. The glomerular layer is pervaded by dendrites from mitral cell neurons, these in turn transmit information to the olfactory bulb that is located in the cerebral cortex.

Specialised receptor cells (olfactory receptor neurons) of the olfactory epithelium in the nose detect smells. Olfaction relies on the binding of odourant molecules to receptors that are located on the receptor cells. Olfaction has complex systems of coding, displaying differing methods for coding the receptor stimulus. There are numerous central projections that allow for the perception and interpretation of important sensory inputs.

Located in the roof of each nostril is the nasal mucosa. It is the nasal mucosa that contains the sensory epithelium – the olfactory epithelium this is covered by mucus. As well as the sensory cells, the epithelium contains Bowman's glands which produce the secretion that saturates the surface of the receptors. This aqueous secretion contains mucopolysaccharides, immunoglobulins, proteins (such lysozyme) and various enzymes.

A pigmented-type of epithelial cell is also located in the nasal mucosa (membrane), the reason for its pigmentation is unknown. The nasal epithelium contains the receptor cells, possessing a terminal enlargement above the epithelial surface, with approximately 8 to 20 olfactory cilia. The cilia do not waft or beat, they contain the smell receptors.

Olfactory nerve and the cribriform plate

Small, unmyelinated axons of the olfactory receptor cells form the fine fibres of the first cranial nerve and travel centrally toward the ipsilateral olfactory bulb making contact with the second-order neurons. The trigeminal nerve (cranial nerve V) sends fibres to the olfactory epithelium detecting caustic chemicals, such as ammonia. The cribriform plate of the ethmoid bone, separated at the midline by the crista galli, comprises a number of small foramina, the olfactory nerve fibres traverse this.

Olfactory bulb

The olfactory bulb lies inferior to the basal frontal lobe and is a highly organised structure composed of several distinct layers and synaptic specialisations. The layers are:
- glomerular layer
- external plexiform layer
- mitral cell layer
- internal plexiform layer
- granule cell layer.

See Figure 55.3.

Olfactory tract

Mitral cell axons project into the olfactory cortex via the olfactory tract. Medial fibres of the tract contact the anterior olfactory nucleus and the septal area. There are some fibres that project to the contralateral olfactory bulb via the anterior commissure.

It is assumed that the thalamic connections serve as a conscious mechanism for odour perception, while the amygdala and the entorhinal area are limbic system components and might be involved in the affective mechanisms of olfaction.

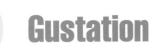

Gustation

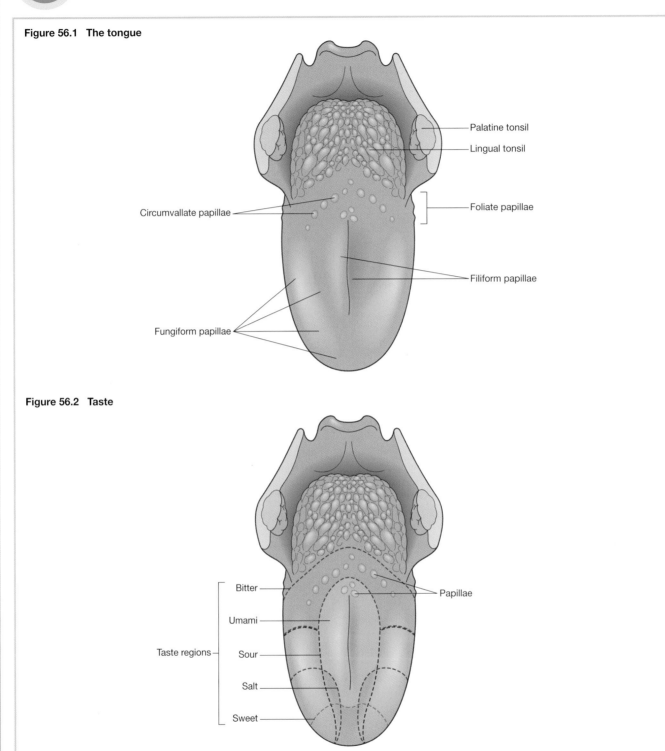

Figure 56.1   The tongue

- Palatine tonsil
- Lingual tonsil
- Foliate papillae
- Circumvallate papillae
- Filiform papillae
- Fungiform papillae

Figure 56.2   Taste

- Bitter
- Umami
- Taste regions
- Sour
- Salt
- Sweet
- Papillae

Gustation

Gustation comes from 'gusto' meaning taste or like, it is the formal term for the sense of taste. In order to create the sensation of taste, a substance has to be in solution of saliva so that that substance can enter the taste pores.

Taste drives the appetite and also protects us from poison. Mostly when we taste bitter or sour this causes dislike because most poisons are bitter, while foods that have gone off taste acidic.

The tongue

The tongue is a muscular organ in the mouth and is covered with moist, pink tissue called mucosa. The papillae give the tongue its rough texture. Thousands of taste buds cover the surfaces of the papillae (see Figure 56.1).

Anatomy and physiology

The taste bud, located on the tongue, is the functional unit that allows us to discriminate between the tastes of sweet, sour, salty and bitter. There are over 100 taste receptor cells in each taste bud.

The sense of taste is mediated by groups of taste buds, these sample oral concentrations of a large number of small molecules and report a sensation of taste to centres located in the brainstem. The papillae are projections of a connective tissue core covered with squamous epithelium. The types of papilla are circumvallate (vallate), foliate, fungiform and filiform (see Figure 56.2).

The taste buds are so small they cannot be seen by the naked eye and a microscope is needed to see them, however, the papillae can be observed by close inspection of the surface of the tongue. The fungiform papillae stand out clearly on a blue background. Taste buds have a life span of about 10–12 days.

As well as signal transduction by taste buds, it is also evident that the sense of smell is profoundly affected by the sensation of taste.

The sense of taste is equivalent to the excitation of taste receptors, and receptors for a large number of particular chemicals have been recognised that influence the reception of taste. These include receptors for such chemicals as sodium, potassium, chloride, glutamate and adenosine. Five categories of tastes are generally recognised, they are:

- salty
- sour
- sweet
- bitter
- umami.

Monosodium glutamate is the taste of umami which has recently been recognised as a unique taste as it cannot be elicited by any amalgamation of the four other taste types. Glutamate is present in a number of protein-rich foods and is particularly abundant in ripened cheese.

The perception of taste appears to be influenced by thermal stimulation of the tongue. For some people, warming the front of the tongue creates a clear sweet sensation and cooling leads to a salty or sour sensation. None of the tastes are elicited by a single chemical.

Taste bud anatomy

Taste buds are made up of groups of about 40 columnar epithelial cells that are bundled together along their long axes. The taste cells within a bud are arranged in such a way that their tips form a small taste pore and through this pore extend microvilli from the taste cells. The microvilli of the taste cells contain taste receptors and it has been suggested that most taste buds contain cells that have receptors for two or three of the basic tastes.

Intertwined among the taste cells in a taste bud is a system of dendrites of sensory nerves that are called taste nerves. When the binding of chemicals to their receptors stimulate taste cells, they depolarise and this depolarisation is spread to the taste nerve fibres resulting in an action potential that is eventually transmitted to the brain. This nerve transmission rapidly adapts; after the first stimulus, a powerful discharge is seen in the taste nerve fibres, however within a few seconds the response reduces to a steady-state level at a much lower amplitude.

When the taste signals are transmitted to the brain, a number of efferent neural pathways are activated, these are important to digestive function. Tasting food, for example, is followed very quickly by increased salivation and also by low-level secretory activity in the stomach.

Taste preferences often change in conjunction with the needs of the body. For example, we like the taste of sugar as we have an absolute need for carbohydrates; we get cravings for salt because we have to have sodium chloride in the diet.

Appendix 1: Cross-references to chapters in *Pathophysiology for Nurses at a Glance*

Chapter in *Anatomy and Physiology for Nurses at a Glance*	Relevant chapter in *Pathophysiology for Nurses at a Glance*
Part 1: Foundations	
1. The genome	All
2. Homeostatic mechanisms	All
3. Fluid compartments	Chapter 7
4. Cells and organelles	Chapter 2
5. Transport systems	Chapter 2
6. Blood	Chapters 16, 17, 18 and 19
7. Inflammation and immunity	Chapter 3
8. Tissues	Chapter 3
Part 2: The nervous system	
9. The brain	Chapters 12, 13, 14 and 15
10. Structures of the brain	Chapters 12, 13, 14 and 15
11. The spinal cord	Chapter 12
12. The blood supply	Chapter 15
13. The autonomic nervous system	All
14. The Peripheral nervous system	All
Part 3: The heart and vascular system	
15. The heart	Chapters 20, 21, 22 and 23
16. Blood flow through the heart	Chapters 20, 21, 22 and 23
17. The conducting system	Chapters 20, 21, 22 and 23
18. Nerve supply to the heart	Chapters 20, 21, 22 and 23
19. Structure of the blood vessels	Chapters 17 and 22
20. Blood pressure	Chapter 7
21. Lymphatic circulation	Chapters 10 and 47
Part 4: The respiratory system	
22. The respiratory tract	Chapters 24, 25 and 26
23. Pulmonary ventilation	Chapter 17
24. Control of breathing	Chapter 6
25. Gas exchange	Chapters 20 and 21
Part 5: The gastrointestinal tract	
26. The upper gastrointestinal tract	Chapters 29 and 31
27. The lower gastrointestinal tract	Chapters 27, 28, 30 and 31
28. The liver, gallbladder and biliary tree	Chapters 32, 33, 34 and 35
29. Pancreas and spleen	Chapter 34
30. Digestion	Chapter 30
Part 6: The urinary system	
31. The kidney: microscopic	Chapters 38 and 39
32. The kidney: macroscopic	Chapters 36, 37 and 38
33. The ureter, bladder and urethra	Chapters 38 and 39
34. Formation of urine	Chapters 36 and 37
Part 7: The male reproductive system	
35. External male genitalia	Chapters 41 and 42
36. The prostate gland	Chapters 40 and 43
37. Spermatogenesis	Chapter 44

Anatomy and Physiology for Nurses at a Glance, First Edition. Ian Peate and Muralitharan Nair. © 2015 John Wiley & Sons, Ltd. Published 2015 by John Wiley & Sons, Ltd.
Companion website: www.ataglanceseries.com/nursing/anatomy

Chapter in *Anatomy and Physiology for Nurses at a Glance*	Relevant chapter in *Pathophysiology for Nurses at a Glance*
Part 8: The female reproductive system	
38. Female internal reproductive organs	Chapter 48
39. External female genitalia	Chapter 45
40. The breast	Chapter 47
41. The menstrual cycle	Chapter 46
Part 9: The endocrine system	
42. The endocrine system	Chapters 49, 50, 51 and 52
43. The thyroid and adrenal glands	Chapters 50 and 52
44. The pancreas and gonads	Chapters 34 and 49
Part 10: The musculoskeletal system	
45. Bone structure	Chapters 53, 54, 55, 56 and 57
46. Bone types	Chapters 53, 54 and 55
47. Joints	Chapters 53, 54 and 55
48. Muscles	Chapters 53, 54, 55, 56 and 57
Part 11: The skin	
49. The skin layers	Chapters 58, 59, 60 and 61
50. The skin appendages	Chapters 58, 59, 60 and 61
51. Epithelialisation	Chapters 58, 59 and 61
52. Granulation	Chapters 58, 59 and 61
Part 12: The senses	
53. Sight	Chapters 67, 68, 69 and 70
54. Hearing	Chapters 62 and 63
55. Olfaction	Chapters 64 and 66
56. Gustation	Chapters 64 and 65

Appendix 2: Normal physiological values

Haematology
Full blood count
Haemoglobin (males) 13.0–18.0 g/dl
Haemoglobin (females) 11.5–16.5 g/dl
Haematocrit (males) 0.40–0.52
Haematocrit (females) 0.36–0.47
MCV 80–96 fl MCH 28–32 pg
MCHC 32–35 g/dl

White cell count 4–11 × 109/l

White cell differential
Neutrophils 1.5–7 × 109/l
Lymohocytes 1.5–4 × 109/l
Monocytes 0–0.8 × 109/l
Eosinophils 0.04–0.4 × 109/l
Basophils 0–0.1 × 109/l

Platelet count 150–400 × 109/l
Reticulocyte count 25–85 × 109/l OR 0.5–2.4%

Erythrocyte sedimentation rate
Westergren Under 50 years:
Males 0–15 mm/1st h
Females 0–20 mm/1st h

Over 50 years:
Males 0–20 mm/1st h
Females 0–30 mm/1st h

Plasma viscosity (25 °C)
1.50–1.72 mPa/s

Coagulation screen
Prothrombin time 11.5–15.5 s
International normalised ratio <1.4
Activated partial thromboplastin time 30–40 s
Fibrinogen 1.8–5.4 g/l
Bleeding time 3–8 m

Coagulation factors
Factors II, V, VII, VIII, IX, X, XI, XII 50–150 IU/dl

Factor V Leiden
Von Willebrand factor 45–150 IU/dl
Von Willebrand factor antigen 50–150 IU/dl
Protein C 80–135 IU/dl
Protein S 80–120 IU/dl
Antithrombin III 80–120 IU/dl
Activated protein C resistance 2.12–4.0
Fibrin degradation products < 100 mg/l
D-Dimer screen < 0.5 mg/l

Haematinics
Serum iron 12–30 µmol/l
Serum iron-binding capacity 45–75 µmol/l
Serum ferritin 15–300 µg/l
Serum transferrin 2.0–4.0 g/l
Serum B12 160–760 ng/l
Serum folate 2.0–11.0 µg/l
Red cell folate 160–640 µg/l
Serum haptoglobin 0.13–1.63 g/l

Haemoglobin electrophoresis
Haemoglobin A > 95%
Haemoglobin A2 2–3%
Haemoglobin F < 2 %

Chemistry
Serum sodium 137–144 mmol/l
Serum potassium 3.5–4.9 mmol/l
Serum chloride 95–107 mmol/l
Serum bicarbonate 20–28 mmol/l
Anion gap 12–16 mmol/l
Serum urea 2.5–7.5 mmol/l
Serum creatinine 60–110 µmol/l
Serum corrected calcium 2.2–2.6 mmol/l
Serum phosphate 0.8–1.4 mmol/l
Serum total protein 61–76 g/l
Serum albumin 37–49 g/l
Serum total bilirubin 1–22 µmol/l
Serum conjugated bilirubin 0–3.4 µmol/l
Serum alanine aminotransferase 5–35 U/l
Serum aspartate aminotransferase 1–31 U/l
Serum alkaline phosphatase 45–105 U/l (over 14 years)
Serum gamma glutamyl transferase 4–35 U/l (<50 U/l in males)
Serum lactate dehydrogenase 10–250 U/l
Serum creatine kinase (Males) 24–195 U/l
Serum creatine kinase (Females) 24–170 U/l
Creatine kinase MB fraction < 5%
Serum troponin I 0–0.4 µg/l
Serum troponin T 0–0.1 µg/l
Serum copper 12–26 µmol/l
Serum caeruloplasmin 200–350 mg/l
Serum aluminium 0–10 µg/l
Serum magnesium 0.75–1.05 mmol/l
Serum zinc 6–25 µmol/l
Serum urate (males) 0.23–0.46 mmol/l
Serum urate (females) 0.19–0.36 mmol/l
Plasma lactate 0.6–1.8 mmol/l
Plasma ammonia 12–55 µmol/l
Serum angiotensin-converting enzyme 25–82 U/l
Fasting plasma glucose 3.0–6.0 mmol/l

Anatomy and Physiology for Nurses at a Glance, First Edition. Ian Peate and Muralitharan Nair. © 2015 John Wiley & Sons, Ltd. Published 2015 by John Wiley & Sons, Ltd.
Companion website: www.ataglanceseries.com/nursing/anatomy

Haemoglobin A1 C 3.8–6.4%
Fructosamine < 285 µmo/l
Serum amylase 60–180 U/l
Plasma osmolality 278–305 mosmol/Kg

Lipids and lipoproteins

The target levels will vary depending on the patient's overall cardiovascular risk assessment.
Serum cholesterol: < 5.2 mmol/l
Serum LDL cholesterol: < 3.36 mmol/l
Serum HDL cholesterol: > 1.55 mmol/l
Fasting serum triglyceride 0.45–1.69 mmol/l

Blood gases (breathing air at sea level)

Blood H + 35–45 nmol/l
pH 7.36–7.44
PaO_2 11.3–12.6 kPa
$PaCO_2$ 4.7–6.0 kPa
Base excess ± 2 mmol/l

Carboxyhaemoglobin

Non-smoker < 2%
Smoker 3–15%

Immunology/rheumatology

Complement C3 65–190 mg/dl
Complement C4 15–50 mg/dl
Total haemolytic (CH50) 150–250 U/l
Serum C-reactive protein < 10 mg/l

Serum immunoglobins

IgG 6.0–13.0 g/l
IgA 0.8–3.0 g/l
IgM 0.4–2.5 g/l
IgE <120 kU/l
Serum β2–micro globulin < 3 mg/l

Cerebro-spinal fluid

Opening pressure 50–180 mm H_2O
Total protein 0.15–0.45 g/l
Albumin 0.066–0.442 g/l
Chloride 116–122 mmol/l
Glucose 3.3–4.4 mmol/l
Lactate 1–2 mmol/l
Cell count ≤ 5 ml-1
Differential:
Lymphocytes 60–70%
Monocytes 30–50%
Neutrophils None
IgG/AlB ≤ 0.26
IgG index ≤ 0.88

Urine

Glomerular filtration rate 70–140 ml/min
Total protein < 0.2 g/24 h
Albumin < 30 mg/24 h
Calcium 2.5–7.5 mmol/24 h
Urobilinogen 1.7–5.9 µmol/24 h
Coproporphyrin < 300 nmol/24 h
Uroporphyrin 6–24 nmol/24 h
Delta-aminolevulinate 8–53 µmol/24 h
5-hydroxyindoleacetic acid 10–47 µmol/24 h
Osmolality 350–1000 mosmol/Kg

Faeces

Nitrogen 70–140 mmol/24 h
Urobilinogen 50–500 µmol/24 h
Fat (on normal diet) < 7 g/24 h

Appendix 3: Prefixes and suffixes

Prefix: A prefix is positioned at the beginning of a word to modify or change its meaning. Pre means "before." Prefixes may also indicate a location, number, or time.

Suffix: The ending part of a word that changes the meaning of the word.

Prefix or suffix	Meaning	Example(s)
a-, an-	not, without	Analgesic, apathy
ab-	from; away from	Abduction
abdomin(o)-	Of or relating to the abdomen	Abdomen
acous(io)-	Of or relating to hearing	Acoumeter, acoustician
acr(o)-	extremity, topmost	Acrocrany, acromegaly, acroosteolysis, acroposthia
ad-	at, increase, on, toward	Adduction
aden(o)-, aden(i)-	Of or relating to a gland	Adenocarcinoma, adenology, adenotome, adenotyphus
adip(o)-	Of or relating to fat or fatty tissue	Adipocyte
adren(o)-	Of or relating to adrenal glands	Adrenal artery
-aemia	blood condition	Anaemia
aer(o)-	air, gas	Aerosinusitis
anaes-	sensation	Anaesthesia
alb-	Denoting a white or pale colour	Albino
alge(si)-	pain	Analgesic
-algia, alg(i)o-	pain	Myalgia
all(o-)	Denoting something as different, or as an addition	Alloantigen, allopathy
ambi-	Denoting something as positioned on both sides; describing both of two	Ambidextrous
amni-	Pertaining to the membranous fetal sac (amnion)	Amniocentesis
an-	not, without	Analgesia
ana-	back, again, up	Anaplasia
andr(o)-	pertaining to a man	Android, andrology
angi(o)-	blood vessel	Angiogram
ankyl(o)-, ancyl(o)-	Denoting something as crooked or bent	Ankylosis
ante-	Describing something as positioned in front of another thing	Antepartum
anti-	Describing something as 'against' or 'opposed to' another	Antibody, antipsychotic
arteri(o)-	Of or pertaining to an artery	Arteriole, artery
arthr(o)-	Of or pertaining to the joints, limbs	Arthritis
articul(o)-	joint	Articulation
-ase	enzyme	Lactase
-asthenia	weakness	Myasthenia gravis
ather(o)-	fatty deposit, soft gruel-like deposit	Atherosclerosis
atri(o)-	an atrium (esp. heart atrium)	Atrioventricular
aur(i)-	Of or pertaining to the ear	Aural
aut(o)-	self	Autoimmune
axill-	Of or pertaining to the armpit (uncommon as a prefix)	Axilla
bi-	twice, double	Binary
bio-	life	Biology
blephar(o)-	Of or pertaining to the eyelid	Blepharoplast
brachi(o)-	Of or relating to the arm	Brachium of inferior colliculus
brady-	'slow'	Bradycardia
bronch(i)-	bronchus	Bronchiolitis obliterans
bucc(o)-	Of or pertaining to the cheek	Buccolabial
burs(o)-	bursa (fluid sac between the bones)	Bursitis

Anatomy and Physiology for Nurses at a Glance, First Edition. Ian Peate and Muralitharan Nair. © 2015 John Wiley & Sons, Ltd. Published 2015 by John Wiley & Sons, Ltd.
Companion website: www.ataglanceseries.com/nursing/anatomy

Prefix or suffix	Meaning	Example(s)
carcin(o)-	cancer	Carcinoma
cardi(o)-	Of or pertaining to the heart	Cardiology
carp(o)-	Of or pertaining to the wrist	Carpopedal
-cele	pouching, hernia	Hydrocele, Varicocele
-centesis	surgical puncture for aspiration	Amniocentesis
cephal(o)-	Of or pertaining to the head (as a whole)	Cephalalgy
cerebell(o)-	Of or pertaining to the cerebellum	Cerebellum
cerebr(o)-	Of or pertaining to the brain	Cerebrology
chem(o)-	chemistry, drug	Chemotherapy
chol(e)-	Of or pertaining to bile	Cholecystitis
cholecyst(o)-	Of or pertaining to the gallbladder	Cholecystectomy
chondr(i)o-	cartilage, gristle, granule, granular	Chondrocalcinosis
chrom(ato)-	colour	Haemochromatosis
-cidal, -cide	killing, destroying	Bacteriocidal
cili-	Of or pertaining to the cilia, the eyelashes; eyelids	Ciliary
circum-	Denoting something as 'around' another	Circumcision
col-, colo-, colono-	colon	Colonoscopy
colp(o)-	Of or pertaining to the vagina	Colposcopy
contra	against	Contraindicate
coron(o)-	crown	Coronary
cost(o)-	Of or pertaining to the ribs	Costochondral
crani(o)-	Belonging or relating to the cranium	Craniology
-crine, crin(o)	to secrete	Endocrine
cry(o)-	cold	Cryoablation
cutane-	skin	Subcutaneous
cyan(o)-	Denotes a blue color	Cyanopsia
cycl-	circle, cycle	
cyst(o)-, cyst(i)-	Of or pertaining to the urinary bladder	Cystotomy
cyt(o)-	cell	Cytokine
-cyte	cell	Leukocyte

Prefix or suffix	Meaning	Example(s)
-dactyl(o)-	Of or pertaining to a finger, toe	Dactylology, polydactyly
dent-	Of or pertaining to teeth	Dentist
dermat(o)-, derm(o)-	Of or pertaining to the skin	Dermatology
-desis	binding	Arthrodesis
dextr(o)-	right, on the right side	Dextrocardia
di-	two	Diplopia
dia-	through, during, across	Dialysis
dif-	apart, separation	Different
digit-	Of or pertaining to the finger [rare as a root]	Digit
-dipsia	Suffix meaning '(condition of) thirst'	Polydipsia, hydroadipsia, oligodipsia
dors(o)-, dors(i)-	Of or pertaining to the back	Dorsal, dorsocephalad
duodeno-	duodenum, twelve: upper part of the small intestine (twelve inches long on average), connects to the stomach	Duodenal atresia
dynam(o)-	force, energy, power	Hand strength dynamometer
-dynia	pain	Vulvodynia
dys-	bad, difficult, defective, abnormal	Dysphagia, dysphasia

Prefix or suffix	Meaning	Example(s)
ec-	out, away	Ectopia, ectopic pregnancy
ect(o)-	outer, outside	Ectoblast, ectoderm
-ectasia, -ectasis	expansion, dilation	Bronchiectasis, telangiectasia
-ectomy	Denotes a surgical operation or removal of a body part. Resection, excision	Mastectomy
-emesis	vomiting condition	Haematemesis
-aemia	blood condition	Anaemia
encephal(o)-	Of or pertaining to the brain. Also see Cerebro	Encephalogram
endo-	Denotes something as 'inside' or 'within'	Endocrinology, endospore
eosin (o)-	Red	Eosinophil granulocyte
enter(o)-	Of or pertaining to the intestine	Gastroenterology
epi-	on, upon	Epicardium, epidermis, epidural, episclera, epistaxis
erythr(o)-	Denotes a red colour	Erythrocyte
-oesophageal, -oesophago-	gullet	Oesophagus
aesthesio-	sensation	Aesthesia

Prefix or suffix	Meaning	Example(s)
ex-	out of, away from	Excision, exophthalmos
exo-	Denotes something as 'outside' another	Exoskeleton
extra-	outside	Extradural haematoma
faci(o)-	Of or pertaining to the face	Facioplegic
fibr(o)	fibre	Fibroblast
fore-	before or ahead	Foreword
fossa	A hollow or depressed area; trenchor channel	Fossa ovalis
front-	Of or pertaining to the forehead	Frontonasal
galact(o)-	milk	Galactorrhoea
gastr(o)-	Of or pertaining to the stomach	Gastric bypass
-genic	Formative, pertaining to producing	Cardiogenic shock
gingiv-	Of or pertaining to the gums	Gingivitis
glauc(o)-	Denoting a grey or bluish-grey colour	Glaucoma
gloss(o)-, glott(o)-	Of or pertaining to the tongue	Glossology
gluco-	sweet	Glucocorticoid
glyc(o)-	sugar	Glycolysis
-gnosis	knowledge	Diagnosis, prognosis
gon(o)-	seed, semen; also, reproductive	Gonorrheoa
-gram, -gramme	record or picture	Angiogram
-graph	instrument used to record data or picture	Electrocardiograph
-graphy	process of recording	Angiography
gyn(aec)o-	woman	Gynaecomastia
halluc-	to wander in mind	Hallucinosis
haemat-, haemato- (haem-,)	Of or pertaining to blood	Haematology
haemangi or haemangio-	blood vessels	Haemangioma
hemi-	one-half	Cerebral hemisphere
hepat- (hepatic-)	Of or pertaining to the liver	Hepatology
heter(o)-	Denotes something as 'the other' (of two), as an addition, or different	Heterogeneous
hist(o)-, histio-	tissue	Histology
home(o)-	similar	Homeopathy
hom(o)-	Denotes something as 'the same' as another or common	Homosexuality
hydr(o)-	water	Hydrophobe
hyper-	Denotes something as 'extreme' or 'beyond normal'	Hypertension
hyp(o)-	Denotes something as 'below normal'	Hypovolemia,
hyster(o)-	Of or pertaining to the womb, the uterus	Hysterectomy, hysteria
iatr(o)-	Of or pertaining to medicine, or a physician	Iatrogenic
-iatry	Denotes a field in medicine of a certain body component	Podiatry, Psychiatry
-ics	organised knowledge, treatment	Obstetrics
ileo-	ileum	Ileocecal valve
infra-	below	Infrahyoid muscles
inter-	between, among	Interarticular ligament
intra-	within	Intramural
ipsi-	same	Ipsilateral hemiparesis
ischio-	Of or pertaining to the ischium, the hip-joint	Ischioanal fossa
-ism	condition, disease	Dwarfism
-ismus	spasm, contraction	Hemiballismus
iso-	Denoting something as being 'equal'	Isotonic
-ist	one who specialises in	Pathologist
-itis	inflammation	Tonsillitis
-ium	structure, tissue	Pericardium
Juxta (iuxta)	Near to, alongside or next to	Juxtaglomerular apparatus
karyo-	nucleus	Eukaryote
kerat(o)-	cornea (eye or skin)	Keratoscope
kin(e)-, kin(o), kinesi(o)-	movement	Kinesthaesia

Prefix or suffix	Meaning	Example(s)
kyph(o)-	humped	Kyphoscoliosis
labi(o)-	Of or pertaining to the lip	Labiodental
lacrim(o)-	tear	Lacrimal canaliculi
lact(i)-, lact(o)	milk	Lactation
lapar(o)-	Of or pertaining to the abdomen-wall, flank	Laparotomy
laryng(o)-	Of or pertaining to the larynx, the lower throat cavity where the voice box is	Larynx
latero-	lateral	Lateral pectoral nerve
-lepsis, -lepsy	attack, seizure	Epilepsy, narcolepsy
lept(o)-	light, slender	Leptomeningeal
leuc(o)-, leuk(o)-	Denoting a white colour	Leukocyte
lingu(a)-, lingu(o)-	Of or pertaining to the tongue	Linguistics
lip(o)-	fat	Liposuction
lith(o)-	stone, calculus	Lithotripsy
log(o)-	speech	
-logist	Denotes someone who studies a certain field	Oncologist, pathologist
-logy	Denotes the academic study or practice of a certain field	Haematology, urology
lymph(o)-	lymph	Lymphoedema
lys(o)-, -lytic	dissolution	Lysosome
-lysis	Destruction, separation	Paralysis
macr(o)-	large, long	Macrophage
-malacia	softening	Osteomalacia
mamm(o)-	Of or pertaining to the breast	Mammogram
mammill(o)-	Of or pertaining to the nipple	Mammillaplasty, mammillitis
manu-	Of or pertaining to the hand	Manufacture
mast(o)-	Of or pertaining to the breast	Mastectomy
meg(a)-, megal(o)-, -megaly	enlargement, million	Splenomegaly, megameter
melan(o)-	black colour	Melanin
mening(o)-	membrane	Meningitis
meta-	after, behind	Metacarpus
-meter	Instrument used to measure or count	Sphygmomanometer
-metry	process of measuring	Optometry
metr(o)-	Pertaining to conditions or instruments of the uterus	Metrorrhagia
micro-	Denoting something as small, or relating to smallness, millionth	Microscope
milli-	thousandth	Millilitre
mon(o)-	single	Infectious mononucleosis
morph(o)-	form, shape	Morphology
muscul(o)-	muscle	Musculoskeletal system
my(o)-	Of or relating to muscle	Myoblast
myc(o)-	fungus	Onychomycosis
myel(o)-	Of or relating to bone marrow or spinal cord	Myeloblast
myri-	ten thousand	Myriad
myring(o)-	eardrum	Myringotomy
narc(o)-	numb, sleep	Narcolepsy
nas(o)-	Of or pertaining to the nose	Nasal
necr(o)-	death	Necrosis, necrotising fasciitis
neo-	new	Neoplasm
nephr(o)-	Of or pertaining to the kidney	Nephrology
neur(i)-, neur(o)-	Of or pertaining to nerves and the nervous system	Neurofibromatosis
normo-	normal	Normocapnia
ocul(o)-	Of or pertaining to the eye	Oculist
odont(o)-	Of or pertaining to teeth	Orthodontist
odyn(o)-	pain	Stomatodynia
-oesophageal, oesophago-	gullet	Oesophagogastrectomy
-oid	resemblance to	Sarcoidosis
ole	small or little	Micromole
olig(o)-	Denoting something as 'having little, having few'	Oliguria

Prefix or suffix	Meaning	Example(s)
-oma (singular), **-omata** (plural)	tumour, mass, collection	Sarcoma, teratoma
onco-	tumour, bulk, volume	Oncology
onych(o)-	Of or pertaining to the nail (of a finger or toe)	Onychophagy
oo-	Of or pertaining to the an egg, a woman's egg, the ovum	Oogenesis
oophor(o)-	Of or pertaining to the woman's ovary	Oophorectomy
ophthalm(o)-	Of or pertaining to the eye	Ophthalmology
optic(o)-	Of or relating to chemical properties of the eye	Opticochemical, biopsy
orchi(o)-, orchid(o)-, orch(o)-	testis	Orchiectomy, orchidectomy
-osis	A condition, disease or increase	Harlequin type ichthyosis, psychosis, osteoperosis
osseo-	bony	Osseous
ossi-	bone	Peripheral ossifying fibroma
ost(e)-, oste(o)-	bone	Osteoporosis
ot(o)-	Of or pertaining to the ear	Otology
ovo-, ovi-, ov-	Of or pertaining to the eggs, the ovum	Ovogenesis
oxo-	addition of oxygen	

Prefix or suffix	Meaning	Example(s)
pachy-	thick	Pachyderma
palpebr-	Of or pertaining to the eyelid *[uncommon as a root]*	Palpebra
pan-, pant(o)-	Denoting something as 'complete' or containing 'everything'	Panophobia, panopticon
papill-	Of or pertaining to the nipple (of the chest/breast)	Papillitis
papul(o)-	Indicates papulosity, a small elevation or swelling in the skin, a pimple, swelling	Papulation
para-	alongside of, abnormal	Paracyesis
-paresis	slight paralysis	Hemiparesis
parvo-	small	Parvovirus
path(o)-	disease	Pathology
-pathy	Denotes (with a negative sense) a disease, or disorder	Sociopathy, neuropathy
pector-	breast	Pectoralgia, pectoriloquy, pectorophony
ped-, -ped-, -pes	Of or pertaining to the foot; -footed	Pedoscope
ped-, pedo-	Of or pertaining to the child	Pediatrics, pedophilia
pelv(i)-, pelv(o)-	hip bone	Pelvis
-penia	deficiency	Osteopenia
-pepsia	Denotes something relating to digestion, or the digestive tract	Dyspepsia
peri-	Denoting something with a position 'surrounding' or 'around' another	Periodontal
-pexy	fixation	Nephropexy
phaco-	lens-shaped	Phacolysis, phacometer, phacoscotoma
-phage, -phagia	Forms terms denoting conditions relating to eating or ingestion	Sarcophagia
-phago-	eating, devouring	Phagocyte
phagist-:	Forms nouns that denote a person who 'feeds on' the first element or part of the word	Lotophagi
-phagy	Forms nouns that denotes 'feeding on' the first element or part of the word	Haematophagy
pharmaco-	drug, medication	Pharmacology
pharyng(o)-	Of or pertaining to the pharynx, the upper throat cavity	Pharyngitis, Pharyngoscopy
phleb(o)-	Of or pertaining to the (blood) veins, a vein	Phlebography, Phlebotomy
-phobia	exaggerated fear, sensitivity	Arachnophobia
phon(o)-	sound	Phonograph, symphony
phos-	Of or pertaining to light or its chemical properties, now historic and used rarely. See the common root **phot(o)-** below	Phosphene
phot(o)-	Of or pertaining to light	Photopathy
phren(i)-, phren(o)-, phrenico	the mind	Phrenic nerve, schizophrenia, diaphragm
-plasia	formation, development	Achondroplasia
-plasty	surgical repair, reconstruction	Rhinoplasty
-plegia	paralysis	Paraplegia
pleio-	more, excessive, multiple	Pleiomorphism
pleur(o)-, pleur(a)	Of or pertaining to the ribs	Pleurogenous
-plexy	stroke or seizure	Cataplexy

Prefix or suffix	Meaning	Example(s)
pneum(o)-	Of or pertaining to the lungs	Pneumonocyte, Pneumonia Pneumatosis, Pneumatic
-poiesis	production	Haematopoiesis
poly-	Denotes a 'plurality' of something	Polymyositis
post-	Denotes something as 'after' or 'behind' another	Postoperation, Postmortem
pre-	Denotes something as 'before' another (in [physical] position or time)	Premature birth
presby(o)-	old age	Presbyopia
prim-	Denotes something as 'first' or 'most-important'	Primary
proct(o)-	anus, rectum	Proctology
prot(o)-	Denotes something as 'first' or 'most important'	Protoneuron
pseud(o)-	Denotes something false or fake	Pseudoephedrine
psych(e)-, psych(o)	Of or pertaining to the mind	Psychology, psychiatry
psor-	itching	Psoriasis
-ptosis	falling, drooping, downward placement, prolapse	Apoptosis, nephroptosis
-ptysis	(a spitting), spitting, haemoptysis, the spitting of blood derived from the lungs or bronchial tubes	Haemoptysis
pulmon-, pulmo-	Of or relating to the lungs.	Pulmonary
pyel(o)-	pelvis	Pyelonephritis
py(o)-	pus	Pyometra
pyr(o)-	fever	Antipyretic

quadr(i)-	four	Quadriceps

radio-	radiation	Radiowave
ren(o)-	Of or pertaining to the kidney	Renal
retro-	backward, behind	Retroversion, retroverted
rhin(o)-	Of or pertaining to the nose	Rhinoceros, rhinoplasty
rhod(o)-	Denoting a rose-red colour	Rhodophyte
-rrhage	burst forth	Haemorrhage
-rrhagia	rapid flow of blood	Menorrhagia
-rrhaphy	surgical suturing	Herniorraphy
-rrhexis	rupture	Karyorrhexis
-rrhoea	flowing, discharge	Diarrhoea
-rupt	Break or burst	Erupt, interrupt

salping(o)-	Of or pertaining to tubes, e.g. fallopian tubes	Salpingectomy, salpingopharyngeus muscle
sangui-, sanguine-	Of or pertaining to blood	Sanguine
sarco-	muscular, flesh-like	Sarcoma
scler(o)-	hard	Scleroderma
-sclerosis	hardening	Atherosclerosis, multiple sclerosis
scoli(o)-	twisted	Scoliosis
-scope	instrument for viewing	Stethoscope
-scopy	use of instrument for viewing	Endoscopy
semi-	one-half, partly	Semiconscious
sial(o)-	saliva, salivary gland	Sialogogue
sigmoid(o)-	sigmoid, S-shaped curvature	Sigmoid colon
sinus-	Of or pertaining to the sinus	Sinusitis
somat(o)-, somatico-	body, bodily	Somatic
-spadias	slit, fissure	Hypospadias, epispadias
spasmo-	spasm	Spasmodic dysphonia
sperma-, spermo-, spermato-	semen, spermatozoa	Spermatogenesis
splen(o)-	spleen	Splenectomy
spondyl(o)-	Of or pertaining to the spine, the vertebra	Spondylitis
squamos(o)-	Denoting something as 'full of scales' or 'scaly'	Squamous cell
-stalsis	contraction	Peristalsis
-stasis	stopping, standing	Cytostasis, homeostasis
-staxis	dripping, trickling	Epistaxis
sten(o)-	Denoting something as 'narrow in shape' or pertaining to narrowness	Stenography
-stenosis	abnormal narrowing in a blood vessel or other tubular organ or structure	Restenosis, stenosis
stomat(o)-	Of or pertaining to the mouth	Stomatogastric, stomatognathic system

Prefix or suffix	Meaning	Example(s)
-stomy	creation of an opening	Colostomy
sub-	beneath	Subcutaneous tissue
super-	in excess, above, superior	Superior vena cava
supra-	above, excessive	Supraorbital vein

Prefix or suffix	Meaning	Example(s)
tachy-	Denoting something as fast, irregularly fast	Tachycardia
-tension, -tensive	pressure	Hypertension
tetan-	rigid, tense	Tetanus
thec-	case, sheath	Intrathecal
therap-	treatment	Hydrotherapy, therapeutic
therm(o)-	heat	Thermometer
thorac(i)-, thorac(o)-, thoracico-	Of or pertaining to the upper chest, chest; the area above the breast and under the neck	Thoracic
thromb(o)-	Of or relating to a blood clot, clotting of blood	Thrombus, thrombocytopenia
thyr(o)-	thyroid	Thyroidism
thym-	emotions	Dysthymia
-tome	cutting instrument	Dermatome
-tomy	act of cutting; incising, incision	Gastrotomy
tono-	tone, tension, pressure	Tonometry
-tony	tension	Tonicity
top(o)-	place, topical	Topical anesthetic
tort(i)-	twisted	Torticollis
tox(i)-, tox(o)-, toxic(o)-	toxin, poison	Toxoplasmosis
trache(a)-	trachea	Tracheotomy
trachel(o)-	Of or pertaining to the neck	Tracheloplasty
trans-	Denoting something as moving or situated 'across' or 'through'	Transfusion
tri-	three	Triangle
trich(i)-, trichia, trich(o)-	Of or pertaining to hair, hair-like structure	Trichocyst
-tripsy	crushing	Lithotripsy
-trophy	nourishment, development	Pseudohypertrophy
tympan(o)-	eardrum	Tympanocentesis

Prefix or suffix	Meaning	Example(s)
-ula, -ule	small	Nodule
ultra-	beyond, excessive	Ultrasound
un(i)-	one	Unilateral hearing loss
ur(o)-	Of or pertaining to urine, the urinary system; (specifically) pertaining to the physiological chemistry of urine	Urology
uter(o)-	Of or pertaining to the uterus or womb	Uterus

Prefix or suffix	Meaning	Example(s)
vagin-	Of or pertaining to the vagina	Vagina
varic(o)-	swollen or twisted vein	Varicose
vas(o)-	duct, blood vessel	Vasoconstriction
vasculo-	blood vessel	Vasculogenic
ven-	Of or pertaining to the (blood) veins, a vein (*used in terms pertaining to the vascular system*)	Vein, Venospasm
ventr(o)-	Of or pertaining to the belly; the stomachcavities	Ventrodorsal
ventricul(o)-	Of or pertaining to the ventricles; any hollow region inside an organ	Cardiac ventriculography
-version	turning	Anteversion, retroversion
vesic(o)-	Of or pertaining to the bladder	Vesical arteries
viscer(o)-	Of or pertaining to the internal organs, the viscera	Viscera

Prefix or suffix	Meaning	Example(s)
xanth(o)-	Denoting a yellow colour, an abnormally yellow colour	Xanthopathy
xen(o)-	foreign, different	Xenograft
xer(o)-	dry, desert-like	Xerostomia

Prefix or suffix	Meaning	Example(s)
zo(o)-	animal, animal life	Zoology
zym(o)-	fermentation	Enzyme, lysozyme

Appendix 4: Glossary

Absorption: The transport of molecules across epithelial membranes into the body fluids

Acinus: Saliva secreting cluster of cells

Acromegaly: Excessive growth due to the production of excessive growth hormone by the pituitary gland

Active immunity: Immunity involving sensitisation, in which antibody production is stimulated by prior exposure to an antigen.

Adenine: One of the four nitrogen-carbon bases of DNA

Adipose cells: Groups of fat cells forming yellow lobules in subcutaneous tissue

ADH: Hormone produced by the hypothalamus and stored in the posterior pituitary gland

Afferent: Conveying or transmitting to

Allergy: Hypersensitivity caused by exposure to allergens, resulting in the release of histamine and other molecules with similar histamine effects

Anaemia: A condition whereby there is a lack of red blood cells

Anterior: In front of

Antibodies: Substances made by the body's immune system in response, for example, to bacteria, viruses, fungus or cancer cells.

Antigens: A substance that when introduced into the body stimulates antibody production.

Anuria: Without the formation of urine

Apnoea: Cessation of breathing

Aquaporins: Transmembrane proteins that aid water reabsorption

Arthralgia: Pain in a joint

Arthroplasty: Surgical replacement of a joint

Aural: Pertaining to the ear

Atrioventricular node: A section of nodal tissue that lies on the right side of the partition that divides the atria, near the bottom of the right atrium

Atrioventricular valves: Collective name of the two valves that lie between the atria and the ventricles

Axilla: The armpit

Axon: Process of a neuron that carries impulses away from the body

Azoospermia: A condition in which there is a lack of spermatozoa in the semen

Baroreceptors: Sensors located in the blood vessels

Bronchodilation: Expansion of the bronchial air passages

Calcitonin: A hormone secreted by the thyroid gland which controls the levels of calcium and phosphorous in the blood

Cancellous bone: Synonymous with trabecular bone or spongy bone, one of two types of osseous tissue forming bones. The other is cortical bone

Cancer: A tumour characterised by abnormally rapid cell division and the loss of specialised tissue characteristics, usually refers to malignant tumours

Capillaries: Tiny blood vessels

Cardiac cycle: The sequence of events that occurs when the heart beats

Cardiac muscle: Muscle of the heart, consisting of striated muscle cells that are interconnected into a mass called the myocardium

Catabolism: The metabolic breakdown of complex molecules into simpler ones, often resulting in a release of energy

Cations: Positively charged ions

Cell membrane: Outer layer of the cell

Cerebrum: The largest anatomical structure of the brain

Cerebellum: Portion of the brain responsible for coordinated and smooth muscle movements

Ceruminous glands: A specialised integumentary gland secreting cerumen, (or earwax) into the external auditory canal

Chemokines: A family of small cytokines, or signalling proteins secreted by cells

Chemoreceptor: A neuroreceptor that is stimulated by the presence of Chemical molecules

Cholinergic: Denoting nerve endings that liberate acetylcholine as a neurotransmitter, such as those of the Parasympathetic nervous system

Chromosome: Mixture of DNA and protein

Chyme: Creamy, semi fluid mass of partially digested food mixed with gastric secretions

Cochlea: The organ of hearing in the inner ear where nerve impulses are generated in response to sound waves.

Conchal surface: A long, narrow and curled bone shelf (shaped like an elongated sea-shell) that protrudes into the breathing passage of the nose

Conjugated bile: formed by the union of two compounds

Corpus: The main body or mass of a structure

Cortex: The outer aspect of an organ, for example

Corticosteroids: Hormones produced by the adrenal gland, consisting of hydrocortisone (or cortisol)

Cryptorchidism: Developmental defect in which one or both testes fail to descend into the scrotum

Cyanosis: A dark blue condition of the skin and mucous membranes caused by oxygen deficiency

Cytoplasm: Fluid found inside the cell

Cytosine: One of the four nitrogen-carbon bases of DNA

Decussation: Crossing over of neurons

Diaphysis: The shaft of a long bone

Diastolic phase: The relaxation phase when the chambers of the heart fill with blood

Diffusion: The passive movement of molecules or ions from a region of high concentration to low concentration until a state of equilibrium is achieved

Digestion: The chemical and mechanical breakdown of food for absorption

Diplopia: Double vision

Diuresis: Excess urine production

Dura mater: The outermost of the three layers of the meninges that surround the brain and spinal cord

Efferent: Conveying away from the centre of an organ or structure

Effector: A muscle, gland, or organ capable of responding to a stimulus, especially a nerve impulse

Electrolytes: An electrolyte is a compound that ionises when dissolved in suitable ionising solvents such as water

Endo: Internal or within

Endocardium: Inner layer of the heart that lines the chambers and the valves

Endocrine: Glands which secrete hormones directly into the bloodstream

Endocytosis: An energy-using process by which cells absorb molecules (such as proteins) by engulfing them

Endometrium: Lining of the uterus

Enzymes: Biological catalysts – catalysts are substances that increase the rate of chemical reactions without being used up

Epinephrine: Adrenaline

Epiphysis: The end segment of a long bone, separated from the diaphysis early in life by an epiphyseal plate, later this becomes part of the larger bone

Anatomy and Physiology for Nurses at a Glance, First Edition. Ian Peate and Muralitharan Nair. © 2015 John Wiley & Sons, Ltd. Published 2015 by John Wiley & Sons, Ltd.
Companion website: www.ataglanceseries.com/nursing/anatomy

Ethmoid bones: A bone in the skull that separates the nasal cavity from the brain

Extracellular matrix: Any substance produced by cells and excreted to the extracellular space within the tissues, serving as a scaffolding to hold tissues together and helping to determine their characteristics

Exocrine: Glands which secrete hormones into ducts

Exocytosis: The process in which the cell releases materials to the outside by discharging them as membrane-bounded vesicles passing through the cell membrane

Filtration: Passive transport system

Follicle: A small secretory cavity, sac, or gland

Ganglia: A group of neuronal cell bodies lying outside the CNS

Gene: A unit of heredity in a living organism

Gingiva: The fleshy covering over the mandible and maxilla through which the teeth protrude within the mouth

Glucagon: A peptide hormone secreted by the pancreas, raises blood glucose levels

Glycogenesis: The formation of glycogen, the primary carbohydrate stored in the liver and muscle cells

Glomerulus: A network of capillaries found in the Bowman's capsule

Gluconeogenesis: The creation of glucose from non-carbohydrate molecules

Glycolysis: The anaerobic breakdown of glucose to form pyruvic acid

Gonad: A reproductive organ, testis or ovary, producing gametes and sex hormones

Guanine: One of the four nitrogen-carbon bases of DNA

Haemopoiesis: A biological process in which new blood cells are formed, which usually takes place in the bone marrow

Hilum: A small indented part of the kidney

Hirsuitism: Excessive growth of body and facial hair, including the chest, stomach and back

Histamine: A compound secreted by tissue mast cells and other connective tissue cells that stimulates vasodilation and increases capillary permeability

Homeostasis: The tendency of an organism or a cell to regulate its internal conditions, usually by a system of feedback controls, so as to stabilise health and functioning, regardless of the outside changing conditions

Hyaline cartilage: A translucent bluish-white type of cartilage present in the joints as well as the respiratory tract and the immature skeleton

Hydrophilic: Water-loving

Hydrophobic: Water-hating

Hypercapnia: A condition where there is too much carbon dioxide in the blood.

Hypoxia: Term used when a cell or tissue is deprived of oxygen

IgA: Antibodies are found in areas of the body such the nose, breathing passages, digestive tract, ears, eyes and vagina

IgD: Antibodies found in small amounts in the tissues that line the chest

IgE: Antibodies found in the lungs, skin, and mucous membranes

IgG: Antibodies found in all body fluids

IgM: The largest antibody

Immunocompetent: Having a normal immune response

Incus: The middle of three auditory ossicles within the middle-ear chamber (anvil)

Inferior: Below

Inferolateral: Located below and towards the side

Insulin: A peptide hormone, produced by beta cells of the pancreas, it regulates carbohydrate and fat metabolism in the body

Ischaemia: Inadequate blood supply to an organ or part of the body, especially the heart muscles

Isthmus: A narrow organ, passage, or piece of tissue connecting two larger parts.

Juxtaglomerular cells: A microscopic structure in the kidney, which regulates the function of each nephron

Keratin: An insoluble protein present in the epidermis and in epidermal derivatives, such as hair and nails

Labyrinth: An intricate structure consisting of interconnecting passages, for example, the bony and membranous labyrinths of the inner ear

Lactation: The production and secretion of milk by the mammary glands

Lacuna: A small, hollow chamber housing an osteocyte in mature bone tissue or a chondrocyte in cartilage tissue

Lamella: Concentric ring of matrix surrounding the central canal in an osteon of mature bone tissue

Lateral: To the side

Lesion: A wounded or damaged area

Libido: Sexual desire

Ligament: A short band of tough, flexible fibrous connective tissue connecting two bones or cartilages, or holding together a joint

Limbic system: Limbic system structures are involved in many of our emotions and motivations, particularly those that are related to survival

Lipogenesis: The process by which simple sugars such as glucose are converted to fatty acids

Locomotion: Movement

Lymphocytes: White blood cells

Lysosyme: Cellular organelles that contain acid hydrolase enzymes that break down waste materials and cellular debris

Macrophages: White blood cells within tissues, produced by the division of monocytes

Mast cell: A type of connective tissue cell producing and secreting histamine and heparin and promoting local inflammation.

Malleus: The first of three auditory ossicles that attaches to the tympanum (the hammer)

Medial: Toward the centre

Medulla: The inner region of an organ or tissue, particularly when distinct from the outer region or cortex (for example, a kidney, an adrenal gland)

Meiosis: A process in which diploid cells become haploid cells, thus ensuring correct number of chromosomes are passed on to offspring

Melatonin: Hormone secreted by the pineal gland, produces lightening of the skin

Menarche: The first menstrual discharge

Meninges: Three layers of tissue that cover and protect the CNS

Metabolism: Sum total of the chemical reactions occurring in the body

Mitosis: A process by which chromosomes are accurately reproduced in cells during cell division

Myocardium: Muscle layer of the heart

Nasal septum: Bony and cartilaginous partition separating the nasal cavity into two portions.

Node of Ranvier: Periodic gap in the insulating sheath (myelin) on the axon of certain neurons that serves to facilitate the rapid conduction of nerve impulses

Norepinephrine: Noradrenaline

Nephron: Functional units of the kidney

Neuromuscular junction: The junction between a nerve fibre and the muscle it supplies

Neurotransmitters: chemical messengers

Olfactory: Pertaining to the sense of smell

Oocyte: A cell in an ovary which may undergo meiotic division to form an ovum

Optic: Pertaining to the eye

Os: Opening

Osteoblast: A bone-forming cell

Osteoclast: A cell that causes erosion and resorption of bone tissue

Osteocyte: A mature bone cell

Osteons: Or Haversian system; the fundamental functional unit of compact bone

Ossification: The process of bone formation

Ovarian ligament: A cordlike connective tissue attaching the ovary to the uterus

Ovulation: The rupture of an ovarian (graafian) follicle with the release of an ovum

Oxytocin: Hormone that stimulates contractions of the uterus during labour

Palpebra: An eyelid

Papillae: Nipple like structure on the tongue that gives it its rough texture

Pericardium: Double layered sac that surrounds the heart

Perilymph: A fluid of the inner ear providing a liquid-conducting medium for the vibrations involved in hearing and equilibrium

Periosteum: A fibrous connective tissue covering the outer surface of bone

Peripheral resistance: The force against blood flow in a blood vessel

Peristalsis: Wave-like contractions that move food through the digestive tract

Phagocytosis: The process of engulfing and ingestion of particles by the cell or a phagocyte such as a macrophage

Pia mater: Innermost layer of the meninges

Pinna: The outer, fleshy portion of the external ear; also known as the auricle

Pinocytosis: Cells drinking water

Polysaccharides: Long carbohydrate molecules of monosaccharide units joined together by glycosidic bonds

Posterior: Behind

Pneumotaxic area: This area is in the pons and is important for regulating the amount of air one takes in with each breath

Pulmonary circulation: A short circulation from the right ventricle to the lungs and back to the heart

Pulmonary ventilation: The process by which gases are exchanged between atmospheric air and the lungs

Raphe: A ridge or a seam-like structure between two similar parts of a body organ; for example, the scrotum

Receptor: A specialised cell or group of nerve endings that responds to sensory stimuli

Renal cortex: The outer most part of the kidney

Renal medulla: The middle part of the kidney

Renal pelvis: The funnel-shaped section of the kidney

Renal pyramids: Cone-shaped structures of the medulla

Ribosomes: Small bead-like structures in a cell, along with RNA, are involved in making proteins from amino acids

Rugae: The folds or ridges of the mucosa of an organ

Sarcolemma: The membrane covering a striated muscle

Sarcoplasm: The cytoplasm of striated muscle cells.

SA node: The pacemaker of the heart

Sebum: An oily, waterproofing secretion of the sebaceous glands

Semicircular canals: Tubule channels within the inner ear containing receptors for equilibrium.

Sensory nerves: Neurones that carry sensory information from the cranial and spinal nerves into the brain and the spinal cord

Serum: Blood plasma with the clotting elements removed

Septum: Dividing wall of the heart

Somatic nervous system: Voluntary motor division of the peripheral nervous system

Spectrin: A cytoskeletal protein that lines the intracellular side of the plasma membrane

Spermatogenesis: The production or development of mature spermatozoa

Sphincter: A ring-like muscle fibre that can constrict

Stapes: The innermost of the auditory ossicles that fits against the oval window of the inner ear (the stirrup)

Superior: Above

Systemic circulation: Flow of blood from the left ventricle to the whole body

Systolic phase: The phase when the chambers of the heart are actively pumping the blood

Tendon: A band of dense regular connective tissue attaching muscle to bone

Thyroxine (T_4): A hormone secreted by the thyroid gland which regulates metabolism

Triiodothyronine (T_3): A hormone secreted by the thyroid gland which regulates metabolism

Thrombocytes: Cells that play a role in blood clotting

Thymine: One of the four nitrogen-carbon bases of DNA

Thymosins: Small proteins present in many animal tissues. So called because they originate from the thymus gland

Trabeculae: A supporting framework of fibres crossing the substance of a structure, as in the lamellae of spongy bone

Tympanic membrane: The membranous eardrum positioned between the external and middle ear

Unmyelinated: Not covered by myelin sheath

Ureter: Membranous tube that drains urine from the kidneys to the bladder

Urethra: Muscular tube that drains urine from the bladder

Vasodilate: Dilation of blood vessels

Vasoconstrict: Constriction of the blood vessels

Visceral: Pertaining to internal organs of the body

Vomer: One of the unpaired facial bones of the skull

White matter: Myelinated nerve fibres

Zygote: A fertilised egg cell formed by the union of a sperm cell and an ovum

Further reading

Gilroy, A.M. (2013) *Anatomy: An Essential Text Book.* Thieme: New York.

Hankin, M., Morse, D. and Bennett-Clarke, C. (2013) *Clinical Anatomy: A Case Study Approach.* McGraw-Hill: New York.

Jenkins, G.W. Tortora, G.J. (2013) *Anatomy and Physiology: From Science to Life*, 3 edn. Wiley: New Jersey.

Martini, F.H. (2012) *Human Anatomy*, 7 edn. Pearson: New York.

Nair, M. and Peate, I. (2015) *Pathophysiology for Nurses at a Glance.* Wiley: Oxford.

Patton, K.Y. and Thibodeau, G.A. (2013) *The Human Body in Health and Disease*, 6 edn. Elsevier: Missouri.

Peate, I. and Nair, M. (2011) (Eds) *Fundamentals of Anatomy and Physiology for Student Nurses.* Wiley: Oxford.

Tortora, G.J. (2013) *Principles of Anatomy and Physiology*, 14 edn. Wiley: New Jersey.

Index

Page numbers in *italics* denote figures, those in **bold** denote tables.